baby
massage

Proven techniques to calm your baby and assist development

Peter Walker

Founder of The Developmental Baby Massage Centre

hamlyn

For my dear friend and teacher, R D Laing

hamlyn

First published in Great Britain in 2011 by
Carroll & Brown Publishers Limited

An Hachette UK company
www.hachette.co.uk

This fourth edition published in 2024 by Hamlyn,
an imprint of Octopus Publishing Group Ltd,
Carmelite House, 50 Victoria Embankment,
London EC4Y 0DZ
www.octopusbooks.co.uk

Distributed in the US by Hachette Book Group,
1290 Avenue of the Americas, 4th and 5th Floors,
New York, NY 10104

Distributed in Canada by Canadian Manda Group,
664 Annette St, Toronto, Ontario, Canada M6S
2C8

ISBN 978-0-600-63829-2

A CIP catalogue record for this book is available
from the British Library.

Printed and bound in China.

10 9 8 7 6 5 4 3 2 1

Commissioning Editor: Louisa Johnson
Project Editor: Constance Lam
Art Director: Nicky Collings
Photography: Jules Selmes
Assistant Production Manager: Lisa Pinnell

All reasonable care has been taken in the
preparation of this book but the information
it contains is not intended to take the place of
treatment by a qualified medical practitioner.

Before making any changes in your health
regime, always consult a doctor. While all the
therapies detailed in this book are completely
safe if done correctly, you must seek professional
advice if you are in any doubt about any medical
condition. Any application of the ideas and
information contained in this book is at the
reader's sole discretion and risk.

Additional Picture Credits:
Alamy Stock Photo: Anna Tolipova 77;
Dreamstime.com: Geargodz 51, Monkey Business
Images 8, 60, Prostockstudio 62, Tom Wang 93;
iStock: key05 61, SDI Productions 90, SelectStock
22, 23, SnowyPhotoStock 50; Shutterstock
Creative: PorporLing 7, Yellow Cat 6.

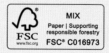

FSC
www.fsc.org

MIX
Paper | Supporting
responsible forestry
FSC® C016973

Foreword

Touch is a universal language that transcends all religions, colours, cultures and creeds. It is your baby's first language, and it is as vital to the health of a baby as any vitamins and minerals.

Foetal responses to touch start in utero at just 12 weeks, and during the last trimester of pregnancy babies are even known to reach out and touch the inside of their mother's abdominal wall when the tummy is rubbed. Following birth, it is through touch that the biological unity between a parent and their baby can continue to function, their skin-to-skin contact being responsible for the regulation of the newborn baby's heartbeat, breathing rhythm and body temperature as well as the flow of milk when breastfeeding.

For the baby, birth is an intense experience. After being pushed, squeezed and sometimes pulled through the birth canal, a soft touch can do much to welcome a baby into this world and relieve any trauma associated with their arrival.

The first 1,001 days of a child's life – from conception to mobility – is recognized as being the most vital time in their development. It is in this primal period that the roots of emotional, physical and physiological health are laid down. The 1,001-critical-days theory recognizes that this early period has a major influence upon child and adult health and future lifestyle choices.

HOW TO USE THE BOOK

- The book is designed to be placed on or next to where you massage your baby so that you can readily refer to the text and pictures for guidance.

- The left-hand page of each exercise explains the purpose and the benefits of the massage, and the right-hand page shows you how to do it, step by step.

- Boxed text highlights any contraindications or important issues to bear in mind while you massage your baby.

As the oldest and the most natural of all the healing arts, baby massage has long been practised to relieve intra-uterine, birth and early-separation trauma. It is used to stimulate and soothe babies and remedy a variety of childhood disorders in many cultures the world over.

Baby massage is an immediate and effective way to develop a loving attachment with your baby. Practising a gentle massage from birth can help parents increase confidence in holding and handling a baby. The techniques and exercises in this book show you how to relieve emotional trauma at every stage. Use them to help secure the full structural health and fitness of your baby through every major postural-motor milestone during those critical 1,001 days.

Baby Massage begins by introducing you to the physical and emotional benefits of massaging your child.

1 **CHAPTER ONE** shows you how to use touches and strokes – with your baby dressed or undressed – in order to develop a close relationship with them in their first few weeks and to help them relax more fully and thrive.

2 **CHAPTER TWO** demonstrates an effective full-body massage routine along with everything you need to know – about the preparation, strokes, oils and ambience – to make it successful. Practised regularly, this toe-to-top routine, along with the early touches, will promote emotional security and the prime physical attributes that constitute good posture, health and fitness. It will enable you to promote and maintain your baby's strength and suppleness. The techniques can also bring to light and alleviate any hidden areas of muscular tension and joint inflexibility.

3 **CHAPTER THREE** shows you how to use massage in later babyhood to help your child to secure and maintain a healthy and comfortable sitting posture.

4 **CHAPTER FOUR** keeps pace with your baby who, as they become more mobile, will want to explore their wide range of physical movement. This is the time to introduce some soft baby yoga, fun and games that engage your baby in versatile movement. These movements are designed to maintain existing suppleness and promote strength, balance and good posture while sitting and standing. At the end of this chapter you also can discover which time is best for you to massage your mobile baby.

5 **CHAPTER FIVE** covers some common complaints and shows how massage and movement can be used to prevent and alleviate these conditions. Additional needs are also discussed, and there is advice on how massage can complement existing forms of treatment and therapy.

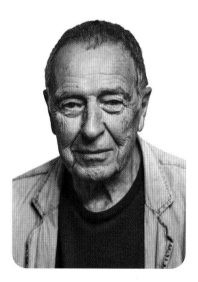

ABOUT THE AUTHOR

PETER WALKER is an international teacher and author. A renowned physical therapist, he has worked with mothers and babies for over 45 years and has been featured in many national publications, including most UK mother and baby periodicals. He has written nine books, some of which have reprinted in over 20 different countries. Peter has also made numerous television appearances and been featured in documentaries and breakfast shows on all UK major channels. His teacher training courses attract professionals from all around the world, and Peter has personally taught and certified some 20,000 teachers.

CONTENTS

The benefits of touch

Touch is the newborn baby's first form of communication. From the first week, placing a hand on their head with a soft cranial touch and/or a gentle massage can do much to relieve intra-uterine and birth trauma. Touch can also relieve the physiological flexion imposed by the womb and stimulate your baby's circulation, breathing and digestive rhythms. As they grow, giving a regular toe-to-top development massage will maintain healthy muscles and joints (see pages 22–49). This can alleviate colic, constipation and some other infant disorders, too.

Emotional benefits

Our muscles relax and tighten in response to our emotions. Developing a loving touch through massage can help your baby to relax and can even ease some tensions associated with separation anxiety. Later, with practice, massage can help with weaning and sleeping.

Massaging your baby:

- Introduces a unique level of confidence and trust to your relationship.
- Brings partners and carers more in touch with their babies – allowing them to strengthen their relationship and learn how to handle their babies with confidence.
- Reduces the circulation of cortisol – a stress hormone in the bloodstream. If massage is done regularly, this reduction is maintained between massage sessions.
- Stimulates the release of the body's natural opiates – endorphins – which subdue pain. Together with the reduction of cortisol, this induces general feelings of wellbeing throughout your baby's body.
- Promotes attachment. As you massage your baby, you maintain eye contact, kiss, caress and vocalize, which encourage closeness in a relationship.

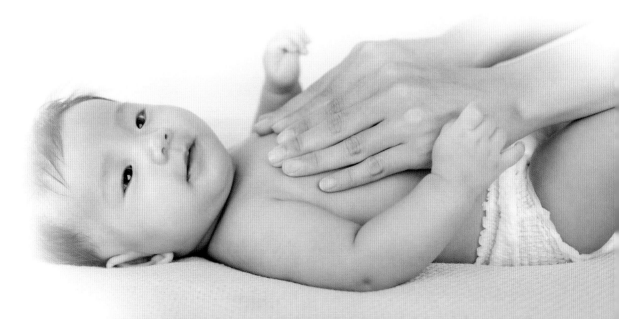

Physical benefits

Our sense of touch allows us to communicate and socially interact with each other. Nowhere is this more apparent than in maternal nursing, where skin-to-skin contact evokes the physiological responses that regulate a baby's vital body rhythms. Including regular massage sessions with your baby conveys emotional, physiological and physical benefits to them. Regular massage produces the following physical benefits:

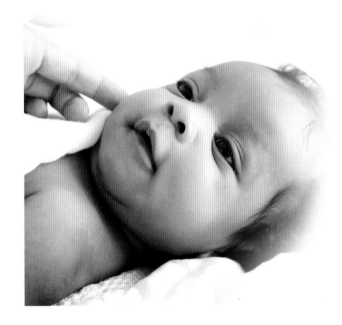

- Healthy growth and development. Touch is every bit as important as vitamins, minerals and proteins; babies who are deprived of touch do not thrive.
- Increases production of growth hormones from the pituitary gland.
- Improves circulation. As muscles relax, they absorb blood and when they contract, they help to pump blood back to the heart and aid the venous return. The periphery of your baby's body – the top of their head and their hands and feet – are often cold because their circulatory system is not fully developed, so massage will warm their hands and feet.
- Helps muscle relaxation and joint flexibility. Massage enables muscles to relax, and as they do so, they allow the free movement of the body's joints. Joint flexibility is vital in enabling your baby to establish a wide range of physical movements and mobility.

- Cleanses your baby's skin and helps to remove dead cells. Massage opens the pores and encourages the elimination of toxins and the secretion of sebum – the natural oil that aids the skin's elasticity and resilience and resistance to infections.
- Stimulates the vagus nerve. One branch of this nerve leads to the gastrointestinal tract, where it facilitates the release of food absorption hormones such as insulin and glucose.
- Promotes the flow of waste-removing lymphatic fluid thus improving the body's resistance to infection.

INTRODUCING YOUR BABY TO MASSAGE

All babies live in the "here and now" and signal their needs as they occur. By establishing close physical contact with your baby from the outset, you can respond to their needs immediately every time.

Human babies are born prematurely compared with other mammals and, although birth is seen as the separation of mother and baby, this is not nature's intention. The nerve connections in a newborn's brain are still developing so a baby retains the emotional–umbilical connection established in the womb. As a primary caregiver you need to maintain this link with your baby.

A vaginal birth gives the baby a powerful massage that stimulates the vital organs to function. Immediately after birth a baby needs to be placed in their parent's arms, so that skin-to-skin contact can regulate their survival systems.

Communication through touch

Although a desire to be held, stroked and touched continues throughout our lives, it is at its most intense in infancy. A newborn baby is far from independent and an extended period of exterogestation – a need to be held outside the womb – is known to have a profound impact on physical, emotional and psychological development. It gives a baby

time to coordinate all their senses in this new and unfamiliar environment with help.

As adults we open our minds and exhale when we wish to "consume" the pleasure of a loving embrace. A clenched fist and a sharp inhalation or "freezing" of the body and breath signals resistance to an unwanted emotional exchange. Likewise a baby's response to sudden movement and stimuli is not an

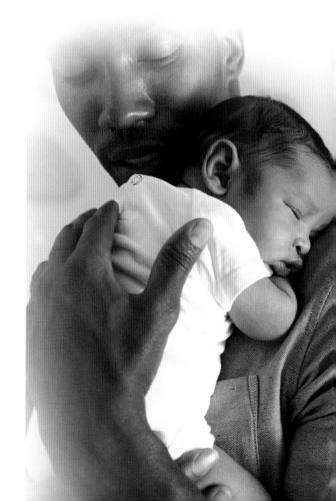

"anxiety reflex" to be ignored, it's a message to the parent to slow down, breathe out and relax, to "be here now" with their baby.

Massaging your baby demands that you are in the "right place" within yourself before you begin. A deep exhalation can relax body and mind. Watch your baby too. Babies breathe with their lower two ribs and abdomen; observing this can show you more than just how to slow down.

Where to start

Give yourself time. Introduce the concepts of this book over your first eight weeks together, choosing quiet, wakeful moments between feeds, with your baby clothed. Centre yourself using exhalation and keep your shoulders relaxed and your hands open. Start by looking at Getting in Touch (see page 10) and read about releasing physiological flexion – this will be especially beneficial if your pregnancy and/or birth was difficult or if your baby was taken to a special care unit following birth.

KEY BENEFITS OF EARLY MASSAGE

- Combined with the benefits of skin-to-skin physical contact, touch triggers the release of "feel-good" hormones to encourage an even closer relationship between you and your baby.

- Massage enables you to get to know your baby in a unique way – it not only strengthens the bond between you, but also satisfies your baby's need for physical contact.

- Baby massage helps parents feel more confident when touching and handling their baby, as well as enabling the infant to feel more secure.

- While allowing parents to get to know their child's structural health, massage also helps maintain a baby's flexibility as they develop. It also encourages abdominal breathing, which not only relaxes the baby, but strengthens the immune system and digestive rhythm.

Getting in touch

In the first days keep your baby close to help them adapt to their new and unfamiliar world. The Tiger in the Tree hold will help you during the more stressful periods (see pages 88–89). But in quieter moments you can quite literally take your baby into the palms of your hands, as shown opposite, as you slowly and gently get the feel of each other. Your baby has been curled tightly in the womb and doing this will help them to let go of the "physiological flexion" that was imposed on them by this position.

You can also re-establish an umbilical connection with your baby. Sit quietly for a moment and feel or connect with your tummy as you breathe out – exhalation – then relax your shoulders and hands.

Breathe out to remain calm so you don't trigger your baby's anxiety reflex. Keep your movements slow. When your baby is happy their tummy will feel soft. If they are upset it will feel hard, like a rock.

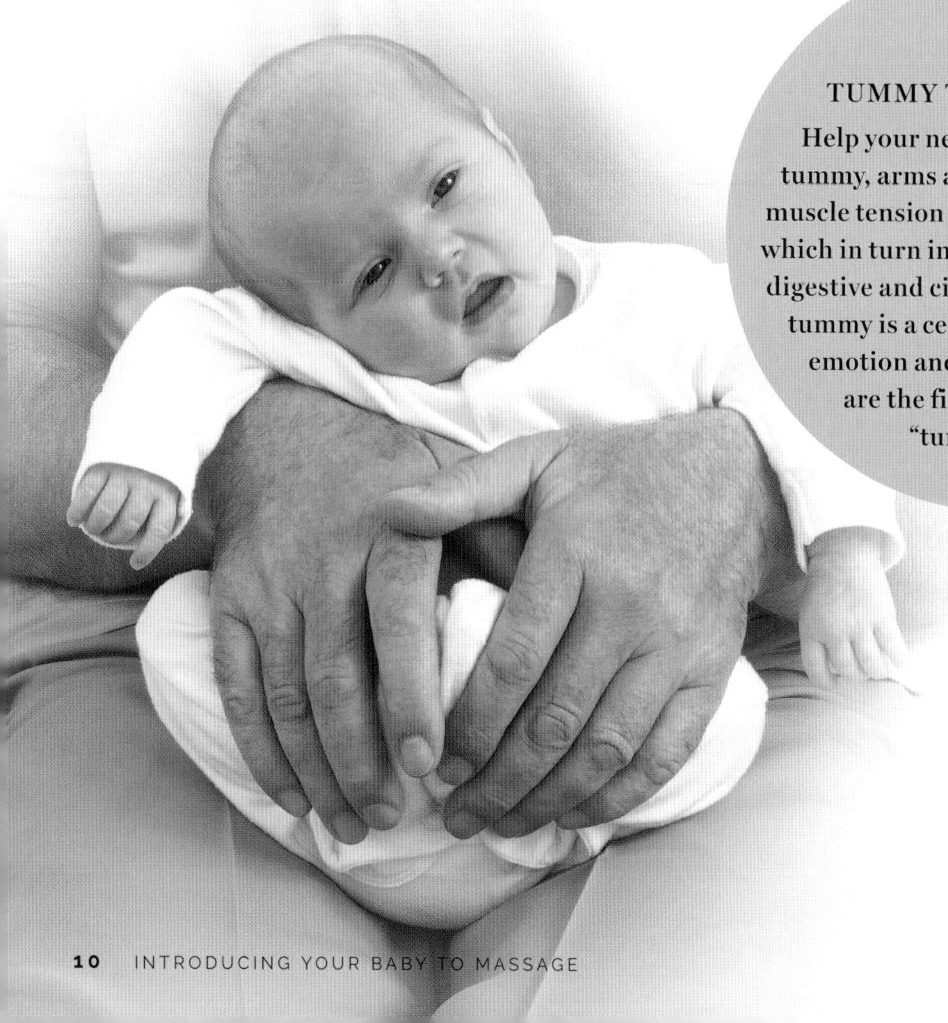

*

TUMMY TRANQUILLITY

Help your new baby to relax their tummy, arms and legs. Releasing the muscle tension evokes a feeling of ease, which in turn improves their breathing, digestive and circulatory rhythms. The tummy is a centre of primal energy, emotion and tranquillity. These are the first steps towards "tummy time".

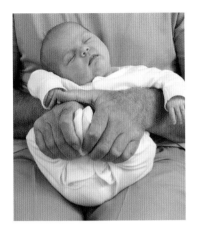

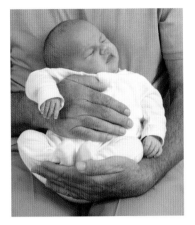

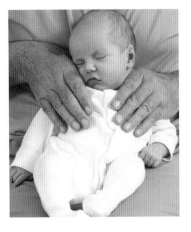

1 Support your baby by letting them lean back against your chest with their bottom resting on your lap. Bring your arms underneath theirs and hold them with their feet together and their knees open.

2 Open one hand to support their lower legs and feet. Place the other hand lightly across their tummy and gently massage it from side to side. Leaning back, slowly remove the hand supporting their legs and feet to encourage your baby to lower their feet, and let them relax and straighten their legs.

NEVER TRY TO FORCE any of the movements. If your baby is not happy with your touches, cradle them in your arms and return to the sequence at another time.

3 Now bring your hands over their shoulders and squeeze softly using relaxed open hands.

4 With relaxed hands stroke gently down the length of their arms to help relax and straighten them. Then gently lay them facing you with their back resting on your thighs and their legs against your tummy – knees open and their feet together – rock them gently.

YOUR BABY MAY FALL ASLEEP as you do this, but if they start to fuss or cry, always stop and give them a cuddle. Remember, massage is something you do with and never to your baby.

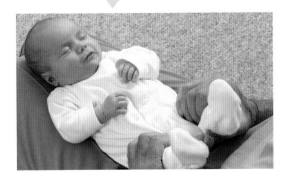

Intro to tummy time

"Tummy time" is the second, and the most important, of your child's motor developmental milestones (see pages 18–19). The belly is a centre of emotion and time spent on the tummy ensures that it can relax fully, allowing for an even deeper breathing rhythm and so an even calmer baby. This is especially important if your baby missed womb time (was premature), they are anxious or were traumatized during labour, delivery or following their birth.

A relaxed abdomen encourages your baby to maintain a deep breathing rhythm, so taking in more oxygen for less effort. This in turn also promotes good circulation and a more relaxed digestive rhythm. Tummy time helps strengthen their back in a way they cannot do in any other natural position. Time spent on the belly will also prevent plagiocephaly, or flat head syndrome.

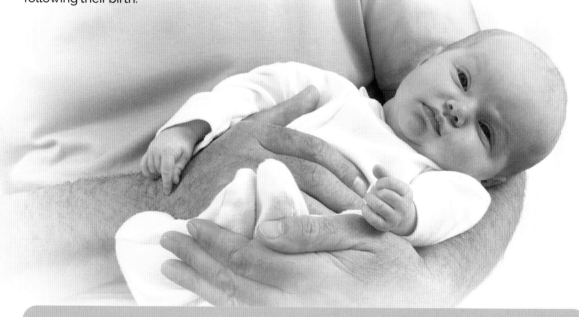

*

DEVELOPING THE STRETCH

Continue to massage your baby's belly as shown on page 11, but now introduce the four easy steps shown opposite to help keep their belly relaxed and prepare them for "tummy time". These techniques help further to stretch open the front of their body on the way to fully releasing the physiological flexion imposed on them in utero, as well as encouraging back strength and spine flexibility.

INTRO TO TUMMY TIME

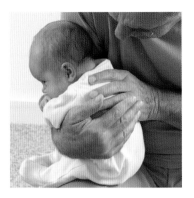

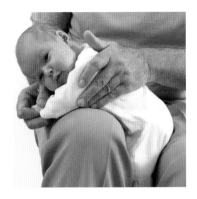

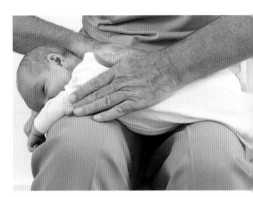

1 Sit in a comfortable chair and place your baby sitting sideways on your lap. Let them lean forwards with their arms extended over your forearm. With relaxed, open hands, gently rub your baby's head and neck, stroking down to the base of their spine and up again.

2 Only when your baby has relaxed in position one, gently lay their tummy forwards over your thighs, with their arms extended and their legs supported between yours. Gently rock your baby and gently rub the sides of their upper back and arms (the latissimus dorsi and trapezius muscles) to relax their arms and shoulders.

3 Only when your baby is relaxed in position two, straighten their legs over your thighs and rock them gently. Now with your baby fully relaxed and extended in this position, stroke down the length of your baby's back and legs, rubbing and patting and rocking them gently.

THIS IS A GREAT FIRST HOLDING POSITION that will allow you to hold your baby while leaving your arms and hands free. (Works a treat at mealtimes.)

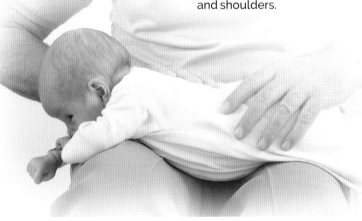

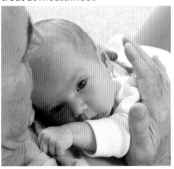

4 Once your baby has fully relaxed, gently slide down on your chair so that your body is inclined. Carefully lift your baby with your hands under their arms and lay them along your chest, in a heart-to-heart position, with their legs extending downwards. Continue to stroke gently down the length of their back.

The sound of your heartbeat will comfort your baby and now that your baby has stretched their tummy, they will be a more relaxed, calmer and happier baby. Include lots of kisses.

Skin-to-skin contact

Once your baby is happy to be stroked while clothed try a little massage with them naked. The techniques opposite provide a good starting point.

First, find a time when -you can be undisturbed for 30 minutes. Check that the room is quiet and not too hot nor too cold. Remove any jewellery and ensure your hands are clean and warm. Lay your baby down on a warm, soft, folded bath towel. Keep your movements slow, follow your exhalation (out breath) and remain centred in your belly, so calm, throughout. You may wish to use one of the oils recommended on page 26 to give you a deeper touch. If you do, carry out the "skin test" on their inner arm first.

Be guided by your intuition. Stop if your baby becomes upset and wrap your baby in the towel to dry when finished.

*

ESTABLISH EYE CONTACT
When face to face with your baby, always maintain eye contact as you touch and stroke them.

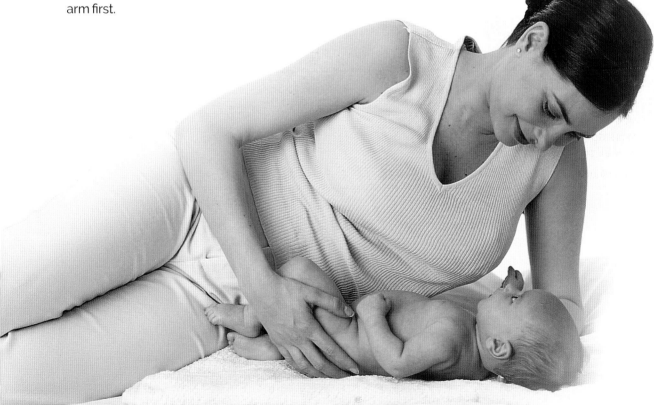

SKIN-TO-SKIN CONTACT

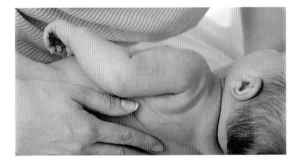

1 Lie down on your left side, with your baby facing you, lying on their right side. Stroke your baby with the whole of your right hand, from the back of their neck to the base of their spine – in the same way as you would stroke a kitten or a puppy.

· Continue for about a minute.

2 Use a circular movement to gently massage around your baby's upper back and then work down the length of their back to the base of their spine.

· Continue for about a minute.

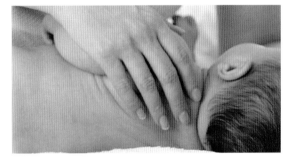

3 Next, slowly take the movement to their arm. Keep your touch gentle and relaxed as you take the stroke from their shoulder to their hand.

· Continue for about a minute.

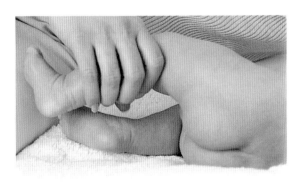

4 Move your hand to the top of your baby's leg and stroke downwards from their hip to their foot with your palm. You can give their leg a little gentle shake to loosen it up and help them to relax.

· Continue for about a minute. Now turn onto your right side and turn your baby to face you. Repeat steps 3 and 4 your baby's right arm and right leg.

Partners and carers

It is very important for partners and carers who did not physically give birth to establish an "umbilical connection" with their new baby in the early weeks.

Your new baby is centred in the "here and now" in the little brain or "enteric nervous system", which is located in the tummy. From here the baby dictates their immediate needs and emotional expressions.

Deepening your exhalation will quieten your mind. It can relax and centre you in your abdomen and bring you more into the "here-and-now" realm of shared feeling. This will also help you to keep your movements slow in order not to trigger your baby's anxiety response.

Starting from birth, follow the techniques described on pages 10–13 with your baby clothed to get more in touch with your child and gain confidence before you follow the steps shown opposite.

You can try this sequence with your baby clothed and, once you are confident with the techniques, move on to massaging with your baby naked. There is no hurry and, if for any reason it's uncomfortable, you can always stop and come back to it when you are both ready.

Learn the Tiger in the Tree carry, too (see pages 88–89), as it is a great way to calm a fractious baby (provided the baby is not hungry).

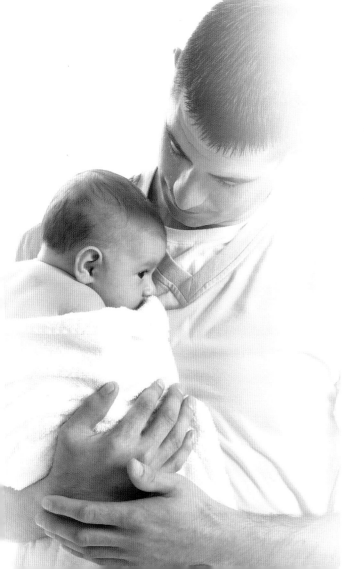

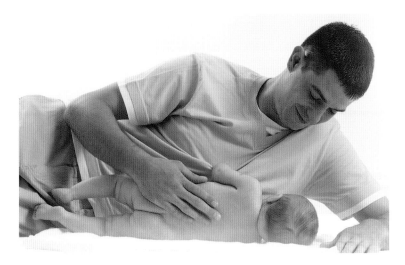

1 Lie down on your side with your baby facing you, lying on their side. Using the relaxed weight of your whole right hand, start stroking your baby's upper back in a circular motion.

TRY AND ESTABLISH EYE CONTACT at the beginning of the massage and maintain it whenever possible throughout.

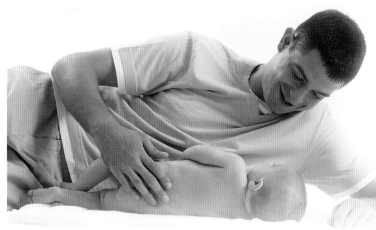

2 Then using the same movement work smoothly right down the length of your baby's spine, to include your baby's lower back.

3 Using the palm of your hand, gently stroke all around the crown of your baby's head in a slow, circular motion.

• Repeat for as long as your baby is relaxed and comfortable.

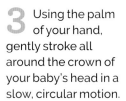

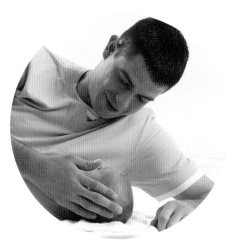

*

Make sure that you are lying comfortably and that your shoulders are relaxed throughout the massage.

Tummy time

This is a very important motor milestone in child development. A baby who experiences ample tummy time from an early age is more likely to crawl – another key developmental milestone that links body and brain development, facilitating sensory integration as well as gross-motor, fine-motor and visual-motor skills.

Tummy time also promotes shoulder stability and core strength. It helps your baby to relax and stretches open the fronts of their thighs, their abdomen, chest and shoulders. In addition the spine can extend, which strengthens the muscles that support it. This in turn helps your child's upright postural development (see also pages 52–55) and is of benefit to their digestive and breathing rhythms, and their immune system. It also results in an even more tranquil disposition.

Many babies resist being placed on their tummies because they are unable to control their head and neck. Their attempts at lifting their head results in them dropping their face forwards to the floor – a painful experience that the child will not wish repeat. Before your baby can lie comfortably (and more safely) on their tummy they need to be able to rest on their elbows. To do this they needs to learn to bring their elbows into line with, or in front of, their shoulders.

Use the steps opposite to prepare your baby. Lay them tummy-forwards on your thighs and, once they are lifting their head and resting on their elbows, lay them on the floor with a rolled towel under their armpits. Once they are totally comfortable in this position you can take away the towel.

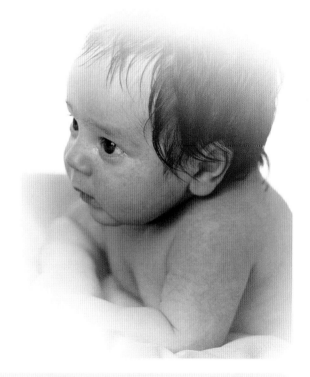

 Do not leave your baby unattended when they are on their tummy, even when your baby can lift themselves onto straight arms. Remove the towel only when your baby can support themselves on their elbows.

TUMMY TIME

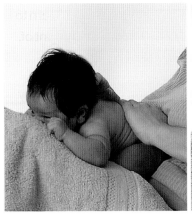 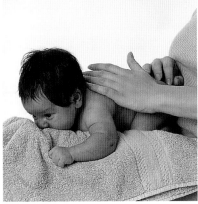 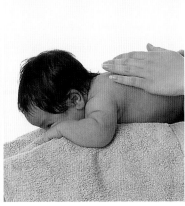

1 Sit comfortably against a wall with your knees bent. Lay your baby belly-down along your thighs, with their knees open.

ENCOURAGE YOUR BABY to straighten their legs, then move your legs from side to side from the hips to rock them gently.

2 Stroke your baby's back, hand-over-hand, and make them feel comfortable in this position, then very gradually lower your knees.

3 Keep bringing your knees down very slowly until your baby is eventually lying flat along your thighs. Keep stroking their back throughout.

4 When your baby is comfortable lying flat, lay them belly-down on a towel on the floor. Support their chest and shoulders on a cushion. Soon you will be able to remove the cushion, giving your baby the full benefits of time on their belly.

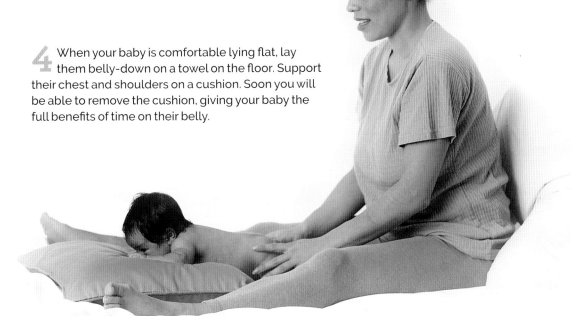

AIR
BATHING

Babies need to spend time naked so that their skin is exposed to fresh air. Known as "air bathing" this is beneficial for maintaining the skin's health and resilience to infection. Once you regularly massage your baby, you will ensure that their skin is consistently air bathed, but even when you are not massaging, you can allow them to spend time naked around the house and, more importantly, outside. By doing this, you are allowing your baby's skin to absorb the life-sustaining and healing properties of oxygen and absorb natural light – major components in the skin's production of vitamin D, which calcifies newly formed bone protein to create stronger bones.

Those times when your baby really isn't ready for, or doesn't fancy, a massage aren't lost if your baby is still given the opportunity to enjoy a greater freedom of movement, unhampered by the restrictions of clothes.

You must make sure that the temperature is comfortable for your naked baby and that they are protected from the sun. If your baby is naked outside, ensure that it is sufficiently warm, with no cool breezes, but that they are out of direct or reflected sunlight. If you are inside, choose a warm, well-ventilated room and keep them away from any draughts. Take care to supervise them at all times.

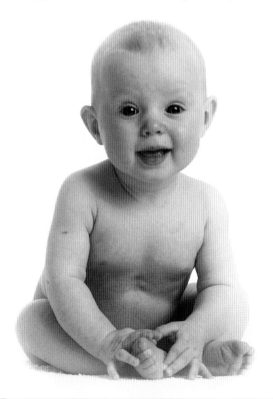

LIGHT THERAPY
From two months, most babies love being naked. Bathing the skin in oxygen and light can help to prevent and cure any minor skin disorders such as nappy rash.

AIR BATHING

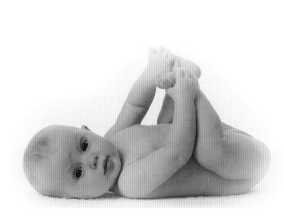

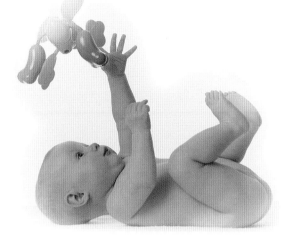

1 Encourage your baby to hold their feet and suck their toes – look at the wonderful range of movement they have.

2 Hold one of their favourite toys above them to encourage them to stretch out their arms and shoulders.

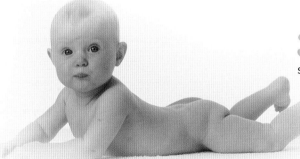

3 Let your baby lie on their belly so that they can stretch out and strengthen their back.

4 Once they are comfortable, they will strengthen themselves even more by pulling their arms and shoulders back.

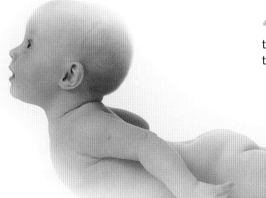

FEET-TO-HEAD MASSAGE

Introducing massage in the early days and weeks will have helped reduce the physiological flexion that kept your baby's arms and legs tucked in towards their body as a newborn. From about eight weeks of age you can introduce a complete toe-to-top-of-head massage.

Most babies prefer massage to begin with their legs and feet and continue up the body, as this is a non-invasive and gradual approach that allows them to get used to the routine. The comprehensive sequence of massage techniques in this section can secure your baby's full structural health and fitness. Starting at your baby's legs and feet also encourages the flexibility of all of their major joints, relaxes their muscles and provides them with a solid foundation for good posture and later mobility.

You do not have to undress your baby until you both feel completely confident. Once your baby is happy to be undressed then try using a massage oil, too (see pages 26–27). Massaging your baby naked will allow you to check their major muscles and joints for any "hidden stiffness" before they strengthen and their range of movement becomes more limited.

Practise the routine regularly – ideally every

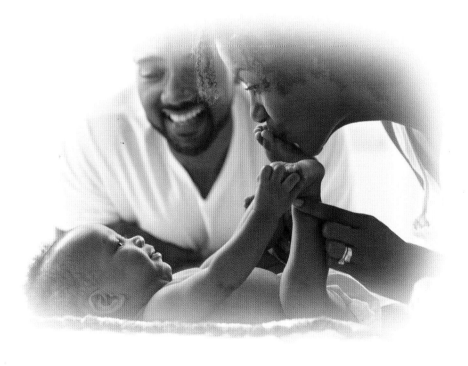

day – to give you and your baby a regular period of special time and closeness. Choose the time of day when they are at their best – not too full, too hungry or too tired. Above all, this is something you do with your baby, not to them, so take your cues from them and punctuate your massage with hugs and kisses.

You do not have to perform the sequence all in one go – you may wish to introduce it a little at a time – but aim to graduate to a full session. The separate massage techniques are designed to interlink, so that all the major muscles and joints are included.

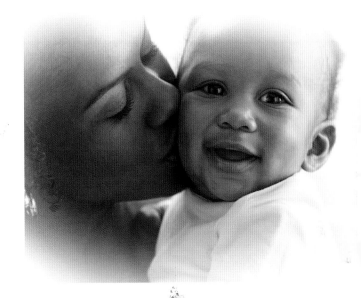

KEY BENEFITS OF FULL-BODY MASSAGE

- Maintains balance and posture through the right order of strength and flexibility.

- Improves muscular coordination and suppleness and relieves muscle and joint inflexibility.

- Releases any hidden areas of tension in muscles and realigns the joints.

- Promotes the flexibility of the spine and strengthens the muscles that support it.

- Aids digestion and tranquillity by allowing the belly to relax more easily.

- Maximizes breathing volume to promote wellbeing; increased oxygen and good circulation will help your baby to thrive.

- Promotes the integrity and alignment of all the major joints and good tone in the muscle groups that control them.

- Cleanses the skin and exposes it to light and oxygen.

BABY MASSAGE STROKES

Your hands are the point of contact between you and your child. If you want your baby literally "in the palm of your hands" while you massage them, first hold them or lay your palms gently on them. Feel them through your palms; your fingers are extensions of your palms. If you begin by touching your baby with your fingertips they may resist you. Stay relaxed and calm and follow your exhalation to stay centred.

As your baby grows and enjoys a more formal massage routine, increase the pressure slightly to give a little more depth to your touch. This gives your baby an important message – they are resilient. The more confident your touch, the more confidence you instil in them. And as your baby develops, you may need to speed up your strokes to hold their attention and keep them engaged.

Punctuate your massage with lots of hugs and kisses and talk and sing to your baby. Babies love to play – this is how they learn best. If you are too serious, your baby will lose interest in the massage and disengage. Keep your hands on your baby's skin. If you stop to turn a page in this book, or to replenish your oil, leave one hand resting upon your baby's body.

HAND POSITION
The way in which you use your hands is very important and will make all the difference to the effectiveness of your baby's massage.

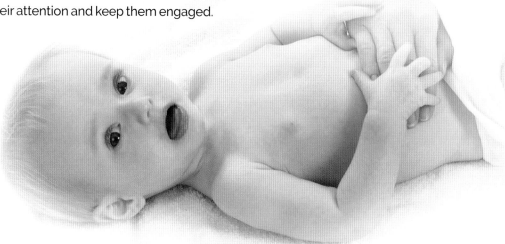

BABY MASSAGE STROKES

The strokes themselves are not difficult to learn and you will soon be doing them intuitively. Rub your hands together and give them a shake to warm them and loosen them up before you start. Keep your hands relaxed from your wrists. The main terms to look out for are as follows:

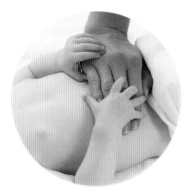

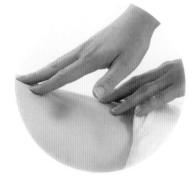

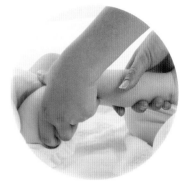

KNEAD
This is a deeper touch that uses the whole hand to press in and massage gently.

STROKE
Move the relaxed weight of your whole hand across the surface of your baby's body.

HAND-OVER-HAND
Begin a movement with one hand as you stop the same movement with the other hand.

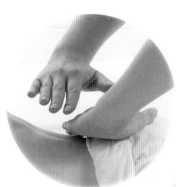

RUB
Press gently and move the relaxed weight of your hand or hands backwards and forwards over your baby's body or limb.

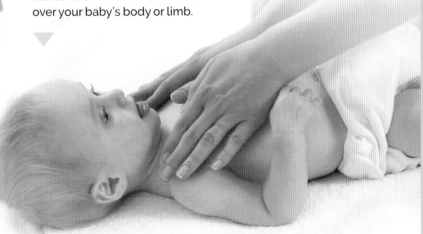

PERCUSSION
Use the relaxed weight of your cupped hands to tap rhythmically on the front or back of the body.

Baby massage oils

Your baby's skin is fine and sensitive, with far more nerve endings than that of any adult. The constant regeneration of healthy cells keeps your baby's skin smooth and moist and a regular massage with an appropriate oil will also cleanse the skin's pores of its dead cells and give it a healthy glow. The oil that you use should allow your hands to glide easily and enable you to give more depth to your touch without discomfort. It should not be highly perfumed nor should it feel too sticky or greasy. It should be pure in its content and whenever possible, organic.

Base oils

Carrier, or base, oils are unperfumed and derived from nuts, seeds and pulp. They often have therapeutic properties on their own – olive oil, for example, is a good moisturizer – but they also can be used to dilute essential oils. Natural fruit or vegetable oils are readily absorbed through the surface of the skin, so you will need to keep replenishing your supply as you massage.

! Always "skin test" the oil you intend to use. Rub a little onto the inner side of your baby's forearm, and wait for one hour to see if there is any allergic reaction. This may look like a heat rash or red blotches, which will disappear after an hour or two. Should this happen, try another oil.

THE FOLLOWING BASE OILS ARE INEXPENSIVE AND WIDELY AVAILABLE

- *Grapeseed* A fine oil, it is known for its purity and easy absorption.
- *Olive* The lighter, yellow olive oil is rich and good for dry skin and cradle cap, and is used extensively in Mediterranean countries.
- *Coconut* A fine oil with a light aroma, widely used throughout the Caribbean.
- *Sunflower* (organic only) A fine, odourless oil, it is highly recommended and can be used with premature babies.

Do not use arachis oil as it is derived from peanuts and your baby may be allergic.

Essential oils

These are highly refined oils that possess the scent and the healing properties of the plant, flower or herb from which they were extracted. They contain natural chemical constituents, which can be used to help promote and maintain health and wellbeing. Each essential oil has unique therapeutic properties. The oils are highly potent, however, and are not recommended for use with very young babies. Before 12 weeks of age, they should not be used at all on your baby (although you can use a recommended base oil). Once your baby is 12 weeks old, oils can be effective, but they should only be used if they are well diluted – two drops of essential oil to three tablespoons of base massage oil. Because your baby is "aroma sensitive", check first that they have no adverse reaction to the blend. Many unexplained episodes of crying are related to highly perfumed oils in aftershaves, cosmetics, household air fresheners and furniture polish. Your baby's sense of smell is what binds them to you. As such it is acutely sensitive.

Not all essential oils are suitable for babies but some of the most useful and effective are:

- *Ravensara* Non-toxic and antiseptic, this is good for viral and skin infections and nappy rash.
- *Chamomile* Calming and soothing, this oil aids digestion and soothes irritability (see page 85). May be helpful for treating colic.
- *Lavender* This antiseptic oil is good for soothing and healing minor burns and bites. It can also be used as a chest or nasal decongestant (see page 79).
- *Eucalyptus* A powerful decongestant, it can be used for a chest-and-back massage (see page 79) to relieve coughs, colds and congestion. Do not use if your baby is having homeopathic treatment.
- *Frankincense* Deeply relaxing with a very pleasant aroma, it can also be used for a chest massage (see page 38) to deepen the breathing rhythm and soothe discomfort. Can promote sleep.
- *Rose otto* Recommended for dry skin, rose otto has a beautiful aroma but it is expensive.

Herbal oils

These are oils created by infusing fresh or dried herbs in a vegetable oil. Ones beneficial to parent and baby are:

- *Arnica* Can help to heal bruising.
- *Lime blossom* Encourages sleep.
- *Calendula* A very healing and soothing oil, it is particularly gentle on skin and can help soothe nappy rash and moisturize dry skin

Using oils

Pour your base massage oil into a saucer so that it is not easily spilled. Make sure that the saucer is within reach, so that you can replenish your oil easily. Dip in your fingers and rub your hands together to spread the oil between your palms and warm it. Reapply when your hands stop gliding smoothly over your baby's skin. Never pour any unused oil back into the bottle, as it may now be contaminated, and do not share your baby's oils.

Buying and storing oils

Choose pure and natural oils, preferably organic, and from a reputable supplier. Essential oils should be packaged in dark coloured glass, since this filters out the sun's ultra-violet light. Choose a cool, dark and dry place to keep oils safely away from heat and inquisitive children. Particularly in summer, carrier and massage oils can benefit by being refrigerated. Before use, you will need to let them stand for a few hours to return to room temperature and give the bottle a shake.

Before you begin

Treat your massage sessions as special times and create a pleasant environment for the massage. Use a quiet, warm, draught-free room in which you can remain uninterrupted for about an hour. If your room is not carpeted, lay a soft towel over a sheepskin or folded blanket for your baby. Your baby will not feel comfortable on a hard surface and, if they lack head control, they could bump their head. If the floor is carpeted, lay your baby on a soft, thick cotton towel; avoid wool as it can irritate your baby's skin. You will need a cushion to sit on and perhaps you and your baby may also find some soft music relaxing.

Have your saucer of massage oil within easy reach and keep a nappy and a fresh towel handy as your baby may pee during the massage. Your baby may well wish to feed after their massage so, whether breast- or bottle-feeding, be prepared.

Relax, enjoy and have fun; massage is meant to be pleasurable for you both. Remain calm and keep your abdominal connection. Keep breathing with your belly. Try not to get distracted or hurried, as this may prevent your baby responding well. If this does happen and your baby gets upset, always stop and give them a feed or a cuddle and then, if you feel inclined, try again – perhaps with them clothed. Babies who resist massage initially are often ones who need it the most and end up most enjoying it.

- Wear comfortable, loose-fitting clothes.
- Wash your hands and make sure that they are not cold; remove any jewellery that could scratch your baby's skin.
- Apply oil as and when necessary, keeping your touch rhythmic.
- Talk and sing to your baby and try to maintain eye contact so that you can be in the "here and now" with your child.
- Always stop if your baby cries. Massage is something that you always do with your baby, never to your baby.

When to massage

Choosing the right time to massage your baby can make all the difference as to whether or not they will enjoy it. A good time to massage your baby is last thing at night, after their bath, or any time during the day when they are at their most

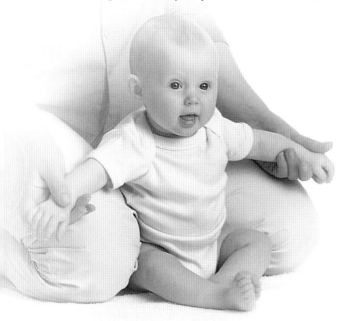

relaxed and responsive. Don't massage them just after a feed; if they are too full, the process can be uncomfortable, especially when you are massaging their belly or laying them on their front to massage their back. Don't massage them when they are hungry either; they are unlikely to tolerate being massaged for any length of time if they are hungry. Try to be consistent with the timing of your massage, so that your baby will learn to anticipate and look forward to the sessions.

If your baby does not immediately seem to respond well to being massaged, persevere – three or four sessions is usually all it takes for babies to begin enjoying it. You do not need to carry out the whole of a sequence in one go; stop when your baby wants to and build your routine little by little each session.

Postures

It is important that you remain relaxed and that your position is comfortable while you are massaging your baby. The sitting positions shown can be fairly easily maintained, but however you sit, make sure that you can lean forwards without straining your back. If you do become uncomfortable at any point during a massage, pause and change your position.

When not to massage

- With the exception of the massages specifically designed to alleviate the symptoms of discomfort (see Chapter Five),

do not massage your baby if they are unwell. In most cases, babies who are feeling ill just want to sleep and be held, but they may respond well to having their feet and/or hands rubbed.

- If your baby is asleep, it is best not to wake them for a massage.
- Do not massage your baby with oil if they have a weeping skin condition, as the oil may exacerbate it. Consult your doctor for advice; they may be able to suggest a suitable alternative.
- If your baby has been immunized, wait for 48 hours to find out how they have been affected. Avoid the site of the injection, but if it leaves a hard lump, you can gently knead it away between your thumb and forefinger once it is no longer sensitive.
- Avoid any areas of your baby's body that are bruised, swollen, inflamed or acutely sensitive. Consult your physician before massaging if you are concerned.

Sit on the edge of a cushion with your legs and feet open in front of you.

Toes and feet

Foot massage is one of the oldest forms of massage and can be extremely relaxing for the whole body. Your baby may find it pleasurable if they are feeling unwell as it can be soothing and it is not obtrusive.

The techniques described opposite will help your baby to open their feet and bring their heels down in preparation for standing – this can be especially helpful if their feet tend to turn inwards. Foot massage can be particularly beneficial for babies with a deformity such as talipes, or club foot (see page 94), where early intervention can help.

Stroking the outer edge of their feet will encourage your baby to extend their heels. Pressing on the sole of the foot while massaging the calf can also encourage the heel to extend. When your baby gets a little older, but before they begin to walk, encourage squatting as this brings the heels down and spreads the toes in preparation for standing.

Once your baby is walking allow them to enjoy the freedom of being barefoot for the first six weeks. Do not encourage your baby to stand on tiptoes for extended periods of time as this shortens the calf muscles, which can affect upright posture.

***

EASY ACCESS

You can massage your baby's feet anywhere you happen to be together and even when they are wearing socks. (Gently massaging your baby's feet while clothed can be non-obtrusive and very soothing if they are unwell.)

TOES AND FEET

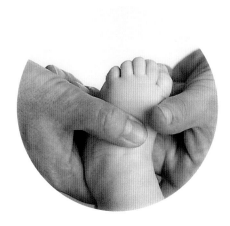

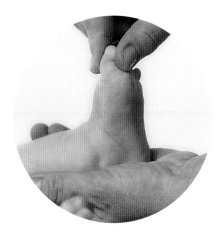

1 Make sure that your hands are well-oiled. Begin to knead and rub the top of your baby's foot with your hands.

· Continue for 2–3 minutes.

2 Then, start to roll each toe between your forefinger and thumb and gently separate the toes so that they fan out slightly.

· Continue for about 20 seconds.

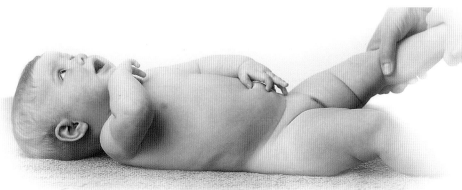

3 Now pull the whole foot smoothly, hand-over-hand, through your palms. You will probably need to replenish your oil at this stage of the massage.

· Continue for about 20 seconds.

4 Flex your baby's ankle and extend the heel by turning their foot outwards with one hand while you rub their calf with the other.

· Continue for about 20 seconds. Repeat with the other foot.

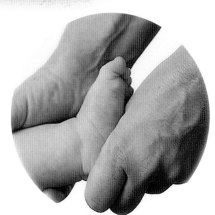

Legs

From about two months, your baby will begin to kick their legs vigorously, bending and stretching them daily for hours on end in a wonderful display of aerobics. This develops the strength and coordination of their postural muscles – the calves, thighs and buttocks – and the flexibility of their hips and knees. The strength and coordination of these muscles and the flexibility of these joints will provide your baby with a strong foundation for upright postures and a wide variety of movement. Both sitting and standing involve balance and this is made far easier when flexible joints provide your baby with a broad base. Your baby will develop the self-confidence to stand tall with the inner feeling that the foundations of their body – their legs – are both strong and flexible.

Massaging your baby's legs will help to promote the development of coordination, strengthen their lower back and maintain the flexibility of their knees and ankles. It will also ensure that there are no areas of hidden tension or stiffness in any of their muscles and joints.

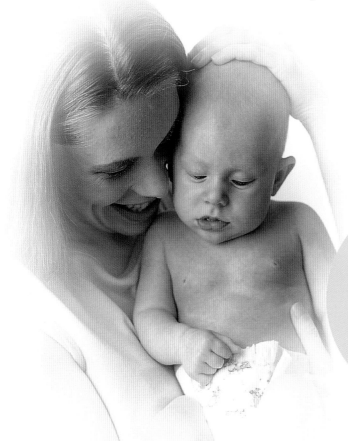

✳

INCREASED FLEXIBILITY
These massage techniques will leave your baby's legs relaxed and supple.

LEGS

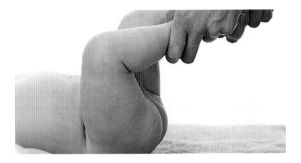 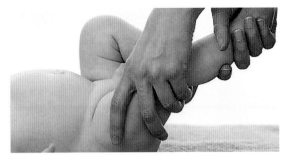

1 Hold both of your baby's legs by the ankles and loosen them up a little by gently "bicycling" them, bending and straightening them alternately.

· Continue for about 20 seconds.

2 Put your left hand at the top of your baby's right leg and pull through your well-oiled palms from their thigh downwards in a hand-over-hand movement, right down to their foot.

· Repeat 4–5 times.

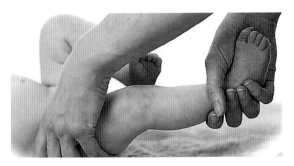

3 Hold your baby's right ankle in your right hand and massage their thigh with your left hand. Massage up the front, then down the back of their thigh.

· Repeat 4–5 times.

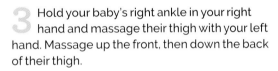

4 Now, pull the whole leg again from the thigh to the foot hand-over-hand.

· Repeat the sequence with your baby's left leg.

5 Shake your baby's legs and rest your hands on their inner thighs. Turn your hands outwards and pull down the back of their knees and calves – they will straighten their legs. Keep gliding your hands up the front and down the back of their legs.

· Repeat 4–5 times.

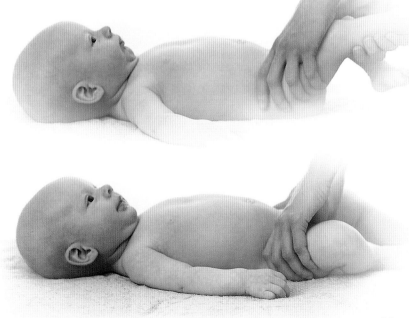

Hips

The flexibility of the hip joints is vital to good posture, both in sitting and standing.

The spine allows very little forwards movement; bending is initiated from the hips. If the hip joints are inflexible then the spine begins to round.

Babies normally enjoy a wide range of hip movement – they can hold their feet and suck their toes effortlessly. When the ability to do this is lacking, or has been lost, a little massage can help restore flexibilty to the hip joints before the muscles really start to strengthen. Practising the massage techniques opposite regularly – at least two or three times a week – will ensure that your baby will enjoy a wide variety of movement and maintain good upright posture, for both sitting and standing, as they develop and strengthen.

Although your baby's hips will have been examined at birth, make sure that they are developing healthily by checking that: they do not "clunk" when they move; they can freely open their knees sideways; both knees look the same when held together and bent; and that the two little creases at the bottom of their spine are uniform when they lie on their belly.

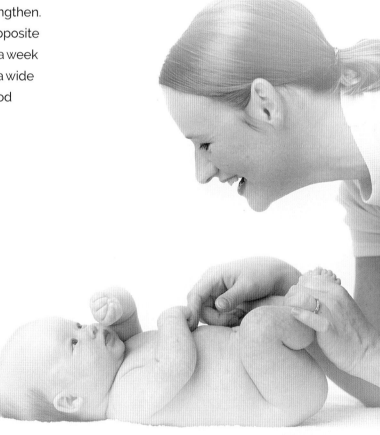

*

PREVENTING HIP INFLEXIBILITY

Babies who practise standing before they are sitting properly are more prone to hip inflexibility. If your baby likes to stand before they are able to sit, practise hip massage two or three times a week.

HIPS

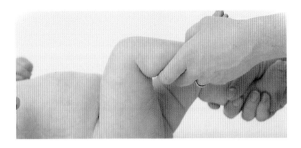

1 Lay your baby on their back and hold their legs by the ankles. Make sure that their legs are relaxed by "bicycling" them a few times – gently bending and straightening them rhythmically one after the other.

• Continue for about 20 seconds.

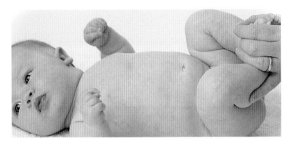

2 Now, clap your baby's feet together and let their knees bend outwards.

• Continue for about 20 seconds.

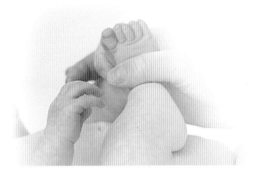

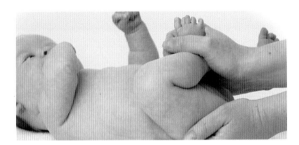

3 Using your right hand, let their knee bend outwards and take your baby's right foot onto their tummy. Hold the foot down gently onto their navel. Keep your right hand in this position while you knead and rub their right buttock and the back of their thigh with your left hand. Do this for about half a minute and then slowly and gently shake your baby's leg straight.

• Repeat the sequence with your baby's left leg.

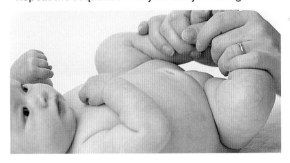

4 Take both of your baby's legs by the ankles and perform a few bicycles. Letting both knees bend outwards, clap the soles of their feet together. Push both of your baby's feet down onto their belly. Gently hold their feet in place with your left hand, place your right hand on their lower back and massage around the base of their spine.

• Continue for about 20 seconds.

5 Gently bend and straighten their legs, and finish by stroking down the front of your baby's legs from the hips to the feet.

• Repeat 4–5 times.

! Be sure to perform the steps in the order they are given. Never force any of the movements and if your baby finds any of the positions uncomfortable, consult your doctor or health visitor.

Belly

Any response to emotion is mirrored by a change in our muscles and nowhere is this more apparent than in the belly, or abdomen – the emotional centre of the body. The tummy muscles tighten in response to fear, anxiety and any other extreme emotions. If you place your hand on your baby's tummy when they are relaxed and happy it will feel soft and malleable; do the same when they are upset and it will be hard and unyielding.

The abdomen is also a centre of tranquillity and massaging your baby's belly, as shown opposite, will help them to relax and become calmer. It can actively relieve infant stress and any traumas associated with birth, as well as help with separation anxiety. A relaxed belly eases digestion, as it allows the diaphragm to move up and down more freely. This not only increases lung capacity and so oxygen intake, but it creates a gentle internal wave that soothes the digestive organs with every breath.

Massaging your baby's tummy can also help to relieve colic and constipation. However, do not massage your baby's tummy if they are upset; try instead Tiger in the Tree (see pages 88–89) – a very special technique for crying babies.

*

TICKLE TREATMENT

If your baby resists having their belly massaged, start by gently patting it, then tickle it to loosen it up, and finally just lay your hand on it briefly. Once your baby accepts this, progress to a full massage.

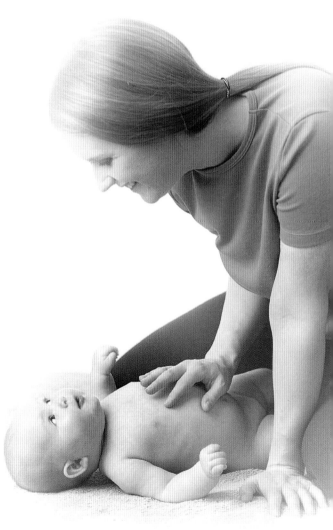

BELLY

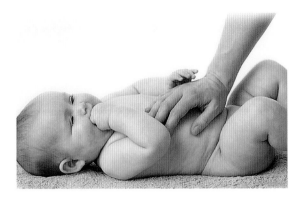

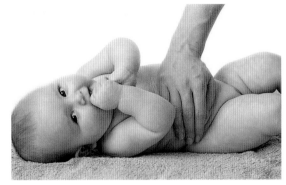

1 Using just the weight of your relaxed hand, massage from your left to your right, in a circular motion. Don't "stroke" the skin, but move your hand and your baby's tummy together, kneading it with gentle and harmoniously clockwise movements.

• Repeat 4–5 times.

2 Place your cupped hand horizontally across your baby's belly and, keeping your hand relaxed, gently knead your baby's tummy from side to side between the lower ribs and the hips. Never push downwards or squeeze the belly hard, as this can cause extreme discomfort.

• Continue for about 20 seconds.

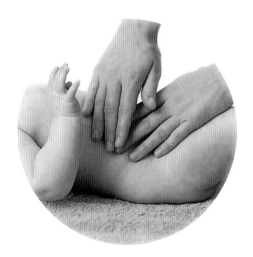

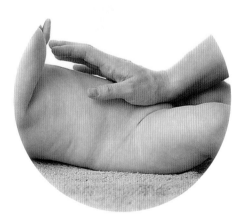

3 Massage hand-over-hand, starting from between the hip and lower ribs on the left side of your baby's body. Work downwards and across to just below the navel. Repeat on the baby's right side.

• Repeat several times on each side.

4 As your baby's tummy relaxes they may release trapped wind. Keep a nappy handy as they might also urinate and, if their stools are loose, they may defecate too. Stay calm if this happens so you don't upset your baby.

Chest

Oxygen is the very spirit of life and the deeper we breathe, the better we feel. As adults, when we receive an emotional or physical shock, we spontaneously take a deep breath or "gasp", and when we are in a state of stress a deep exhalation (out breath) will enable us to calm down. This not only helps us to relax but it also deepens our inhalation (in breath), ensuring the cells of our bodies receive a plentiful supply of oxygen.

Your baby's abdominal breathing rhythm is intuitively healthy – their lower ribs and belly expand on the in breath as they fill their lungs with air and they contract in harmony as their empty them. Your young baby will start to breathe more deeply as they stretch open their chest, arms and shoulders and begin to strengthen and straighten their back in preparation for upright postures and mobility. You can encourage them to maintain their

healthy breathing rhythm and reap the benefits of abdominal breathing. An open chest and a relaxed breathing rhythm will sustain your baby's growth and development and help them to resist and recover from illness and infection. A massage will encourage your baby to maintain their healthy breathing rhythm and enjoy the benefits of a relaxed tummy.

Muscular tension in the chest and tummy can result from repressed or prolonged crying. By mobilizing your baby's chest and ribcage through massage, you enable them to breathe more deeply and efficiently, to gain more oxygen with less effort.

*

IMPROVED BREATHNG

A regular chest massage will help to open your baby's chest and shoulders.

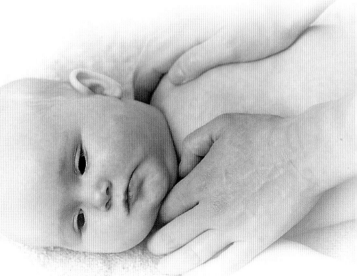

CHEST

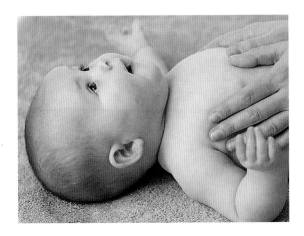

1 Sitting comfortably, with your baby lying on the floor in front of you, place your relaxed well-oiled hands on the centre of your baby's chest.

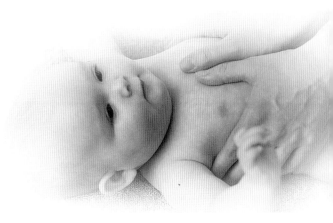

2 Now, with relaxed open hands, massage downwards and outwards around the lower ribcage and return your hands to the centre.

• Repeat 4–5 times.

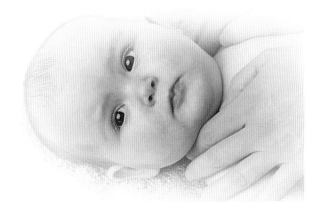

3 Place your hands on the centre of your baby's chest and massage upwards and outwards over their shoulders and return you hands to the centre again.

• Repeat 4–5 times.

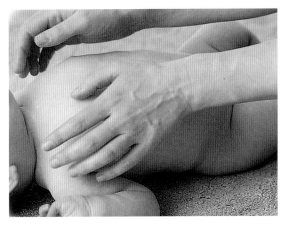

4 Cup your hands and tap them lightly across the top and around the sides of your baby's chest in a percussion movement.

• Continue for about 20 seconds.

Shoulders and arms

A newborn baby keeps their arms folded and tucked into their chest or against the sides of their body. During the normal course of development, they will open their arms first downwards, then outwards and finally upwards. The outwards movement opens and relaxes the shoulders and chest, while simultaneously closing and strengthening the upper back from both sides. Stretching upwards and lifting the arms and hands above the head takes a little longer. This opens the chest from end to end and strengthens the muscles and ligaments around the spine.

If you have followed the previous chapters and your baby is enjoying tummy time, their arms and shoulders should now be stronger and more relaxed. But, if they are still stiff, massage the arms gently from the shoulders, encouraging them downwards, then give the arms a gentle shake. Once your baby can relax their arms in this position, open them outwards to both sides and shake the arms very gently again. Now return to page 13 to help your baby raise their arms and relax even more. If your baby is enjoying tummy time, massage their arms, working upwards above their head. Give the arms a very gentle shake and now roll them onto their tummy to continue to massage their back.

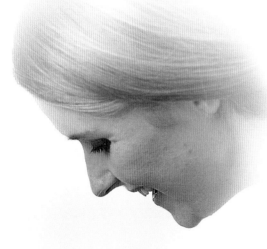

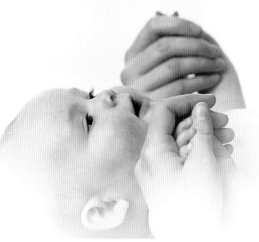

*

LOOSENING UP BABY'S HANDS

You do not have to break the sequence of your massage to work on your baby's hands (see pages 42–43). Arm and hand massage is fun and can be done at any time with or without massage oil.

SHOULDERS AND ARMS

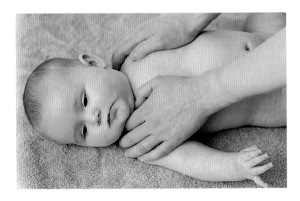

1 Lay your baby on their back in front of you and, with well-oiled hands, work from the top of your baby's chest, moving your hands upwards and outwards over their shoulders and back to the centre.

• Continue for about 20 seconds.

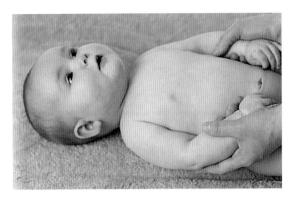

2 Move your hands up and outwards over your baby's shoulders and gently pull their arms downwards – in line with their body – through the centre of your palms. Keeping in contact with their skin, glide your hands back to the top of their chest.

• Repeat 4–5 times.

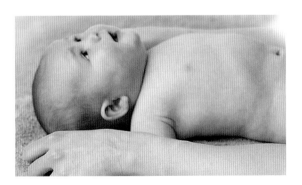

3 Working from the top of their chest, move your hands outwards over your baby's shoulders. Gently and smoothly pull their arms outwards in line with their shoulders. Glide your hands back to the top of their chest. Only when your baby is completely comfortable with these first three steps can you progress to step four.

• Repeat 4–5 times and kiss and blow on your baby's chest.

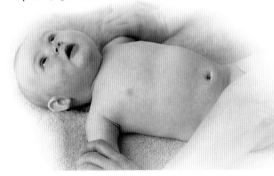

4 Place your hands around the sides of your baby's chest, under their arms, and gently pull their arms upwards through your palms, so that they are above your baby's head. Keep your hands on your baby and glide them lightly back to their chest.

• Repeat 4–5 times.

 You can encourage your baby to open their arms outwards by clapping their hands together very quickly before opening them to make it into a little game.

Hands

Our hands are the most wonderful "organs" of perception. When we speak of our sense of touch, it is associated almost exclusively with our hands. So much of the quality of our everyday lives depends upon the skillful use of our hands and we use them in a variety of ways – for holding, creating and communicating.

Most of our sense of touch in fact comes through the activities that we perform using our fingers. However, to give and receive depth of feeling we use the palms of our hands together with our fingers, and a relaxed exhalation (out breath).

A newborn baby holds their hands and fingers clenched and it can take a few months before they can fully relax them enough to open them at will. Massaging your baby's hands will encourage this development and can be mutually pleasurable. You can do it any time you are sitting together as it is unobtrusive. Hand massage can be done with or without oil, too. Always aim for a light touch and gently shake the hands loose from the forearm.

*

REACHING AND GRASPING

The desire to hold objects, which manifests when your baby stares intently at their hands, is apparent long before they have the skill to reach out and grasp something.

HANDS

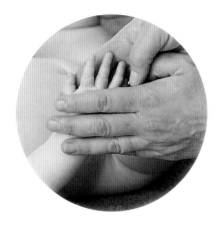

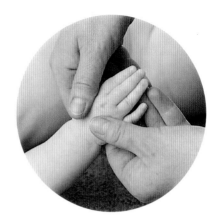

1 Start by opening your baby's hand and rubbing it between your palms.

· Continue for about 20 seconds.

2 Now, relax their hand further by massaging their palm and the back of their hand with your thumbs and index fingers. Work from the wrist to the fingers, squeezing gently backwards and forwards.

· Repeat 3–4 times.

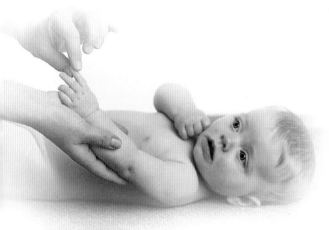

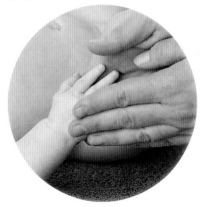

3 Spread your baby's fingers and thumb and, one by one, gently pull each of them through your thumb and forefinger.

· Continue for about 20 seconds.

4 Now rub their whole hand again – back and front – through your palms.

· Repeat the whole sequence with your baby's other hand.

 If you use oil for this massage, make sure it is digestible, organic and non-aromatic, like sunflower or grapeseed, and wipe your baby's hands when you have finished; babies are always sucking on their fingers.

Back and spine

Feeling comfortable in this tummy-forward position is your child's first major postural motor milestone (see pages 18–19). It enables your baby to relax and strengthen in a way that they cannot do in any other natural position. They naturally stretch open their chest and relax the front of their body. It encourages their spine to become flexible and strengthens the muscles and ligaments that support it.

Your baby learns to do this through repeated practice over several weeks. Step by step, they will lift their head, chest, shoulders, arms and legs from the floor, eventually attaining a vital postural motor milestone known as "swimming".

Massaging your baby as they move through this natural phase of development will ensure that their back and spine are both strong and flexible. This not only ensures excellent posture and a well-balanced body but it will also stretch the front of their body, to maintain a relaxed tummy and their natural abdominal breathing rhythm.

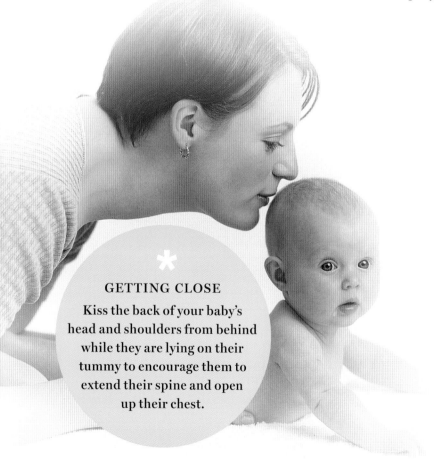

!

Only use this technique when your baby is able to lift their own head, chest and shoulders up from the floor in a tummy-forward position with both arms straight or lifted. Do not try to pull your baby up in this position – your baby must lift up themselves when they are ready.

*

GETTING CLOSE

Kiss the back of your baby's head and shoulders from behind while they are lying on their tummy to encourage them to extend their spine and open up their chest.

BACK AND SPINE

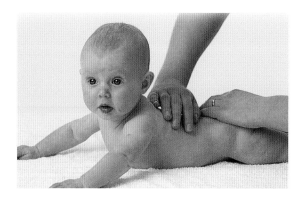

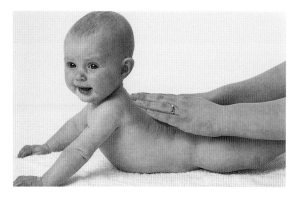

1 Rub plenty of oil into your hands. As your baby lies on their tummy, massage hand-over-hand down their back – from their shoulders down the length of their spine. Use long, firm strokes, but keep your hands relaxed and make it fun for your baby, maybe giving them a tickle now and again!

• **Repeat 4–5 times.**

2 Cup your hands slightly and pat your baby quite firmly all over their back and shoulders, and up and down the entire length of their spine. Everyone loves a pat on the back and your baby is no exception!

• **Continue for about 20 seconds.**

3 When your baby can rest their weight on straight arms, you can develop the massage. Put one well-oiled hand on the centre of your baby's chest, and draw it back across the front of their left shoulder and down their arm a couple of times. Make sure to keep their arm alongside their chest and to take their hand to their hip; do not lift it up for them.

• **Repeat with their right arm.**

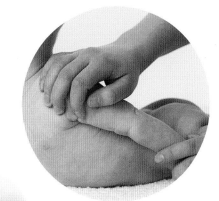

4 Place both of your hands on the front of your baby's chest and gently pull their shoulders back to open their chest. Follow this movement through to pull their arms back, in line with their body, through the centre of your palms, and release gently. Your baby will remain in this position on their own accord before bringing their arms forwards again.

• **Repeat 3–4 times.**

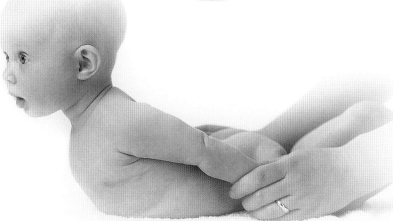

Head and neck

Head and neck massage can be very calming and deeply relaxing for a baby. It can be instantly soothing and is unobtrusive. You can do it almost anywhere and at any time. No prior preparation is needed: your baby can be dressed or undressed and you do not need to use any massage oil. The crown of a baby's head fits perfectly into the palm of your hand and because you always need to support the head when you hold a baby it is easy to include a gentle massage when you cuddle them.

Many babies come into this world with lumps, bumps, bruises and abrasions from blunt force (for example, forceps) and/or emotional trauma. Wait for any obvious signs of injury to abate before you massage the head. When you are both ready, prepare your baby by laying your hand on their head to test their response. Once your baby accepts, massage their head as directed. If your baby had a difficult delivery or if they became "stuck" in the birth canal, practise head massage once or twice a day for as long as you feel they need it.

! If you use oil for this massage, make sure that you wipe your baby's brow to prevent the oil from entering their eyes, as it may temporarily blur their vision. (Used regularly, olive oil can be effective for treating cradle cap.)

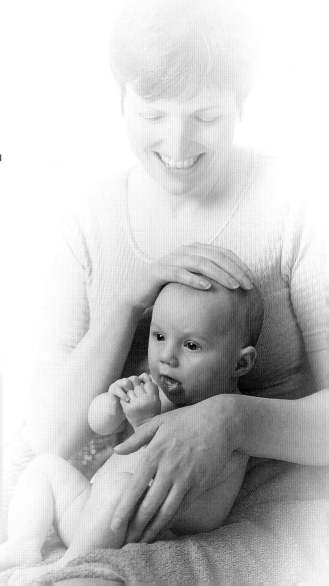

BEFORE YOU BEGIN
Sit comfortably. Let your neck and shoulders go and use your exhalation to relax. If your baby's birth was difficult follow this with a craniosacral massage, see page 48.

HEAD AND NECK

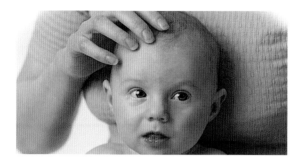

1 Start by lightly massaging around the top of your baby's head in a circular direction with the tips of your fingers.

· Continue for a minute or two.

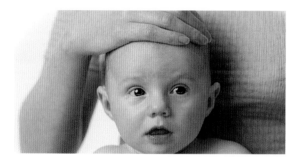

2 Then, stroke all around the crown of your baby's head in a circular direction using the relaxed weight of your palm and fingers.

· Continue lightly for a minute or two.

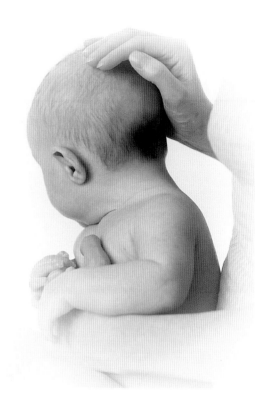

3 Now, using the relaxed weight of your whole hand, stroke all around the back of your baby's head, using a circular motion.

· Continue for about a minute.

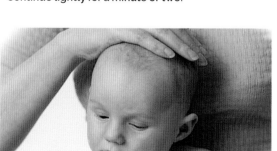

4 Continue the movement to include all of your baby's head. Stroke from the back of their head to the brow and around the crown.

· Continue for as long as you like.

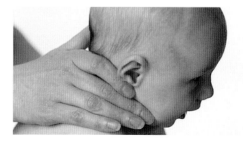

5 Now stroke down the back of your baby's neck and shoulders and gently massage the back of their neck with your fingertips.

· Continue for a minute or two.

CRANIOSACRAL TECHNIQUE

If your baby had a long labour or a difficult delivery – especially if forceps or ventouse were needed – this is a good technique to help them recover. Before you practise this technique, prepare your baby (see pages 46–47) to ensure that they are happy to have their head touched and gently massaged.

The pressure on the baby's head required to open the birth canal can compress the neck and shoulders. The phrenic nerve, a major nerve that passes motor information from the brain to the diaphragm, arises from the back of the neck. If the function of this nerve is impinged it affects the movement of the diaphragm. Releasing this allows the diaphragm to descend deep into the belly with every breath, which can make for a far happier baby with a deeper breathing rhythm.

You need to choose the right moment to practise craniosacral technique – the best time being when your baby is completely relaxed and happy. You may also need another person to assist but, with or without an additional set of hands, the emphasis is on physical alignment of the head and neck and relaxation of the neck and shoulders.

*

BEFORE YOU START
Always check with your doctor before carrying out this technique if your baby is having regular unexplained episodes of distress.

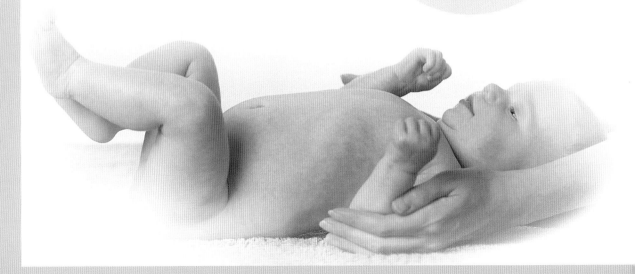

CRANIOSACRAL TECHNIQUE

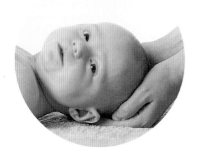

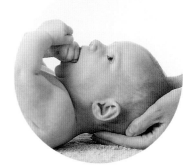

1 Lay your baby gently on their back in front of you, with the crown of their head towards you. Sit behind them and, with your hands open and relaxed, slip your palms under the base of your baby's head and rest them on the floor like a pillow.

2 Gently position your baby's head so that it is perfectly centred, with their chin tucked into their chest to relax and lengthen the back of their neck. Hold your baby's head in this way for about a minute.

3 Once your baby is completely comfortable with step 2, ask your partner, a friend or a family member to help you to extend the technique. While you gently hold your baby's head as above, let your helper sit opposite you and hold your baby's feet. Keeping them together, slowly bend your baby's knees to a right angle, with the soles of their feet facing your helper to ensure that their back is aligned.

· Continue for about 20 seconds.

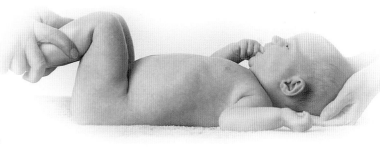

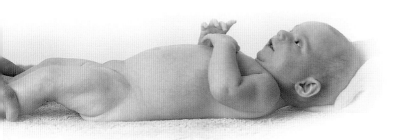

4 Keep holding your baby's head as your helper gently shakes your baby's legs straight before stroking them lightly down the front from their hips to their feet. Let your helper talk, sing and kiss your baby to fully engage them as they do this.

· Continue for about 20 seconds.

SECURING YOUR BABY'S POSTURE

The stages of motor development are universal and, like the development of intelligence, each stage depends upon achieving the previous one. For example, your baby must learn to lie on their tummy and lift themselves off the ground before they can crawl, and then stand before they can walk. The age at which a baby achieves any of these milestones has no bearing upon their intellectual potential. Some babies sit late and walk early, while others sit early, crawl early then walk late. What is important is that your child is not hurried through these stages – they need the time to achieve their full potential at each and every stage of their postural-motor development.

Sitting properly is an art, a major accomplishment for all young babies, and like all the other stages of development, your baby should not be pushed into it nor hurried through it. There is no prescriptive time span on sitting, so take your cues from your baby. Your aim is to help them to secure this part of their development – to massage them through it so that they have the healthiest and most comfortable posture they could wish for.

Continuing to massage your baby can become a challenge once they are sitting on their own. They may no longer be content to lie down for their massage now that they have achieved this stage of development. You will need to work with them to accommodate their changing positions so that they continue to reap the benefits of a comprehensive massage.

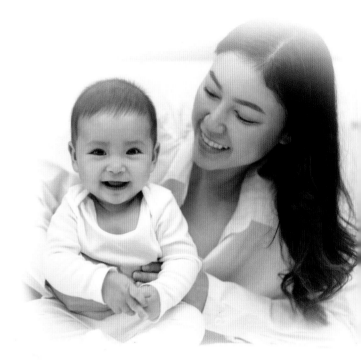

KEY BENEFITS OF SEATED MASSAGE

- Accomplishes a comfortable and healthy posture.

- Maintains abdominal breathing.

- Aids digestion.

- Promotes free and easy movement of the spine in all forward directions.

- Consolidates your baby's posture and helps them to develop confidence in sitting alone.

- Enables you to accommodate your baby's increasing mobility by modifying your techniques.

Helping your baby to sit

During their early weeks, your baby's muscles are not strong enough to support their head and neck and any attempt to pull them into a sitting position will result in them dropping their head forwards and rounding their back. This is an uncomfortable and unhealthy posture that weakens the spine and can inhibit breathing and digestion, so it is best avoided.

By two to three months, having practised tummy time (see pages 18–19), your baby should have developed enough head, neck and back strength to start to sit. Once they can lie on their belly and hold their head up in line with their chest, they are ready to start the preliminary stage of sitting – with your help.

To sit comfortably for any period of time, your baby's hip joints must be flexible enough to allow them to sit on the back of their legs and lean forwards. This position enables free movement of the spine in all forward directions. It also permits their chest to remain open to accommodate a deeper breathing rhythm and their belly to remain relaxed so as not to inhibit the rhythms of digestion.

Do not pull your baby up into a sitting position by their hands. Their wrists will not form properly for some years yet and you will also increase the curvature of their back.

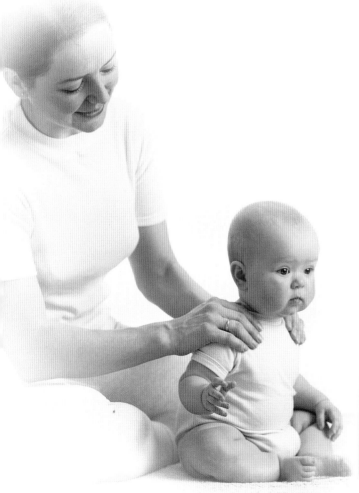

*

STRONG STRAIGHT BACK
To assist your child to sit up straight in this, their first independent sitting position, first encourage them to lean slightly forwards so they sit on the backs of their thighs rather than on the backs of their hips and spine.

HELPING YOUR BABY TO SIT

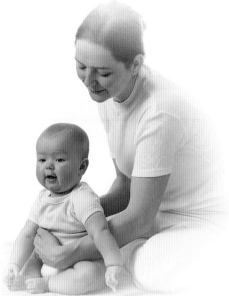

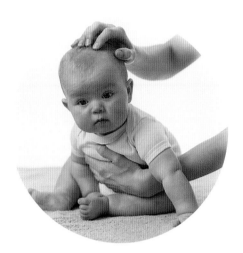

1 Support your baby in a sitting position – with their feet together and their knees open (this is known as the "tailor pose"). Kneel behind them and place one hand around their chest so that they can lean forwards into your palm for support, while taking their weight on the backs of their legs.

2 Now, with the fingertips of your other hand, gently stroke the crown of your baby's head from front to back to relax them.

• Continue for about 20 seconds.

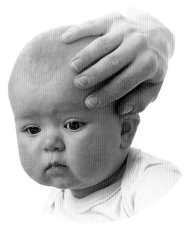

3 Relax your hand, and, using your palm, massage gently all around the crown and sides of their head.

• Continue for about 20 seconds.

4 While still supporting the chest with one hand, use the relaxed weight of your other hand to gently push the back of the hips down towards the floor to "ground" your baby. This will encourage them to transfer their weight downwards onto the back of their thighs, which in turn elongates their spine, promoting a healthy posture.

• Continue for about 20 seconds.

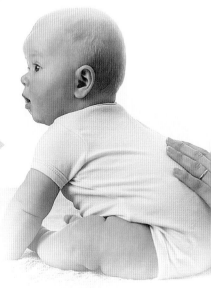

Sitting supported

Your baby will gain strength spending some waking time in the belly-forwards (tummy-time) position. You will know when they are ready to progress to sitting unsupported when they can lie on their belly and support themselves on their arms and hands.

If they try to sit unsupported at this stage, they could fall backwards, forwards or sideways so, before you start, make sure that they are protected on all sides, with cushions if necessary. Sit your baby in the "tailor pose" sitting position – with their feet together and their knees open. Place a long pillow or cushion over their legs, and cushions on each side to enclose them in a triangle. Lean them forwards over the lap cushion – the emphasis is on positioning them so that they can push themselves up straight. Pull their bottom out slightly to ensure they are sitting on the backs of their legs.

Never leave your baby unattended when they are sitting up with the support of cushions.

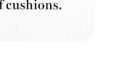

SITTING SUPPORTED

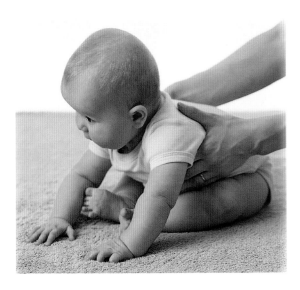

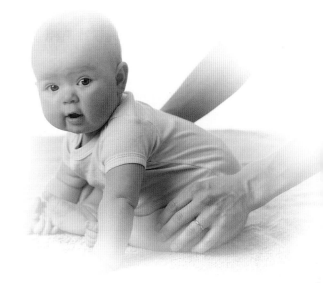

1 Once your baby can support themselves, take away the surrounding cushions and let them lean forwards so that they are supporting their trunk on straight arms, for as long as they are comfortable. Support them by holding them lightly around the waist or hips.

2 Now withdraw support from their back: move your hands downwards and rest your relaxed hands over your baby's legs to "ground" them as they get their balance. Leave their arms free to support themselves. Practise this regularly until you feel they are confident and secure in this position.

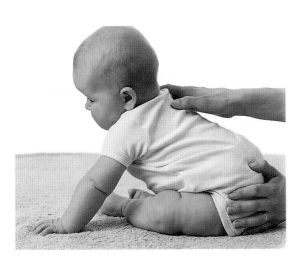

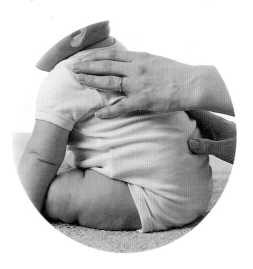

3 Once your baby is secure in this position you can begin to include massage. Steady them with one hand and massage downwards on the back of their hips with your other hand to help them secure their balance.

4 Follow this by massaging hand-over-hand down their back from their shoulders to their lower back, still gently pushing the back of their hips and the base of their spine downwards.

Sitting unsupported

Sitting unsupported is usually achieved at around six or seven months of age. When your baby is fully secure with sitting on their own, they will be able to counterbalance their weight and reach for their favourite toys, take a cup or biscuit and stretch their arms up to you to be lifted. Massage can help your baby to strengthen their "roots" and consolidate their posture. This will give them more confidence when they are sitting independently.

This is an important time for your baby, so don't hurry them onto the crawling stage. Practice will help them to perfect these postures and they are developing the skills that will last them a lifetime. They will know when they have practised enough to move on. If their hips are flexible enough, when they are ready, they will pull themselves over their feet and onto their tummy ready to crawl, then push back onto their knees into the second sitting position.

*

EXTRA SUPPORT
By kneeling with your baby in between your legs, you can offer them support – should they require it – as they learn to sit alone.

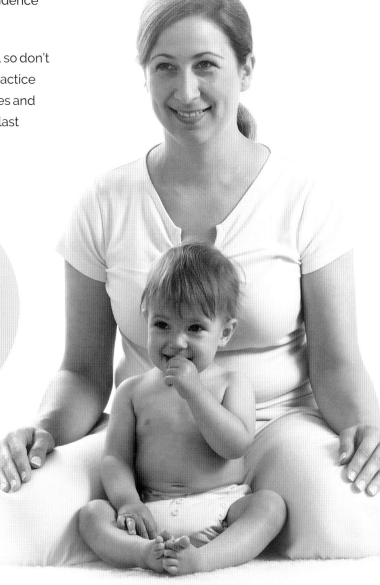

SITTING UNSUPPORTED

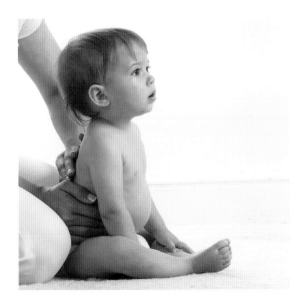

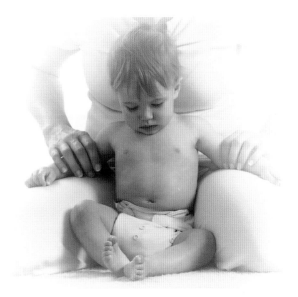

1   As your baby sits, kneel behind them and stroke down their back, hand-over-hand, and around the hips and tops of their legs.

• Continue for about 20 seconds.

2   Stroke over their shoulders and gently pull their arms through your relaxed palms downwards and sideways. This will help relax their arms and shoulders in this position. You may want to use oil here, so that your hands glide easily and you do not pull them off balance.

• Continue for about 20 seconds.

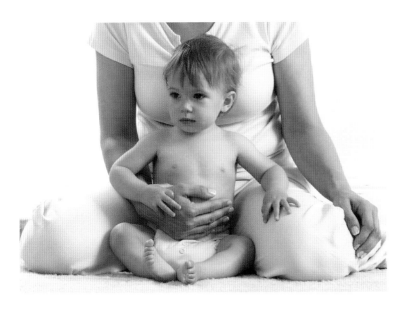

3   Now, provided that your baby's belly is not full, massage their tummy from side to side, by kneading gently with a cupped hand between the ribs and the hips.

• Continue for about 20 seconds.

Second sitting position

When your baby has mastered the tailor pose and pulled themselves forwards onto their hands and knees, they may spend some time pulling forwards and then rocking back into the tailor pose. But soon they will bring their knees together and then sit back between their feet in the second sitting position. This is an easy foundation for making the transition from sitting to crawling and your baby may now start to prefer this sitting position to the tailor pose.

You will have to choose the right moment to massage your baby once they can sit in this position, because once they get mobile, they will not want to remain still for very long.

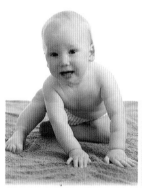
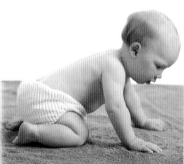
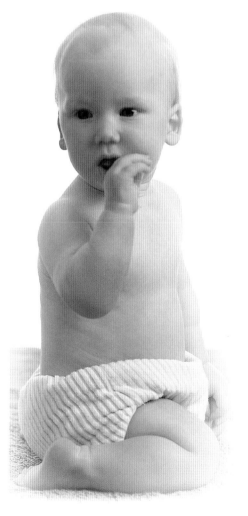

KEEP YOUR BABY'S FEET TURNED INWARDS

! It is important that you do not let your baby sit with their feet turned outwards in a W position as this will make their knees "loose" and can dislocate their hips.

SECOND SITTING POSITION

1 Sitting behind your baby, massage the front of their thighs – from the knees to the hips – stroking backwards and forwards with oiled, relaxed hands. This will relax their front thighs.

• Continue for about 20 seconds.

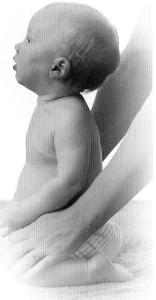

2 Now try to encourage your baby to lean back towards you at about a 30-degree angle. This will help to further relax the front of their thighs and will keep their lower back straight and strong.

• Continue for about 20 seconds.

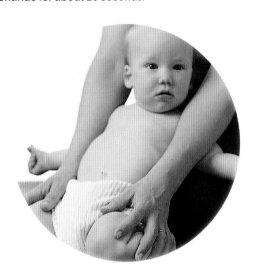

3 Let your baby sit up straight again. Cup your hand slightly and, to relax your baby's belly, stroke from right to left with a circular movement. This can also aid their digestion.

• Continue for about 20 seconds.

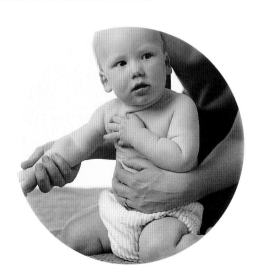

4 Using oil, place your relaxed hands over your baby's shoulders and pull their arms gently and smoothly outwards through the centre of your palms to help them relax their arms and shoulders in this position.

• Continue for about 20 seconds.

MOBILITY
AND SOFT GYMNASTICS

Once your baby is able to sit independently, they will begin moving out of their first sitting position. As they move from sitting to crawling, they will develop their second sitting position and go on to squat, stand and walk. Having created a wide range of versatile movements, your baby will now start to strengthen rapidly and in carrying and moving their ever-increasing body weight from place to place, they will become a little "weightlifter". The more body weight they lift, the stronger your baby will become and, like all weightlifters, unless they continue to make expansive movements, they will lose some of their flexibility as they strengthen and consolidate their body's range of movement.

As your baby starts to crawl, squat, stand and walk, they will no longer wish to stay still for a structured massage, but the following soft gymnastic techniques allow you to continue to positively influence their development while

they are on the move. They can be used for fun and games while maintaining good posture and all-round structural fitness as your baby grows. And they will enable you to continue engaging your baby on a one-to-one basis, to share lots of love and affection.

Like massage, these soft gymnastic games should never be forced or practised against your child's will, and you do not have to do all of the stretches in one go.

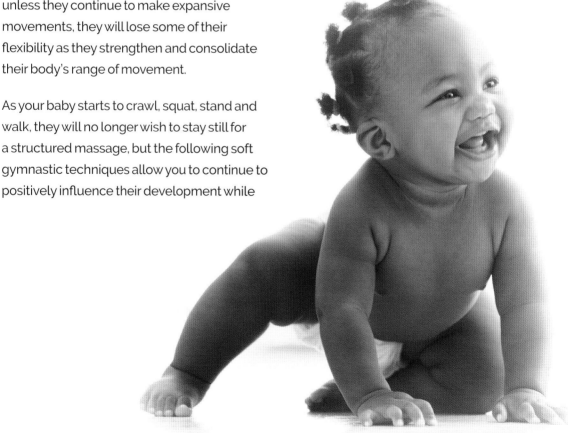

It is better to try them one at a time until you are completely confident and your baby anticipates and enjoys them. You can then aim to fit them in once or twice a week.

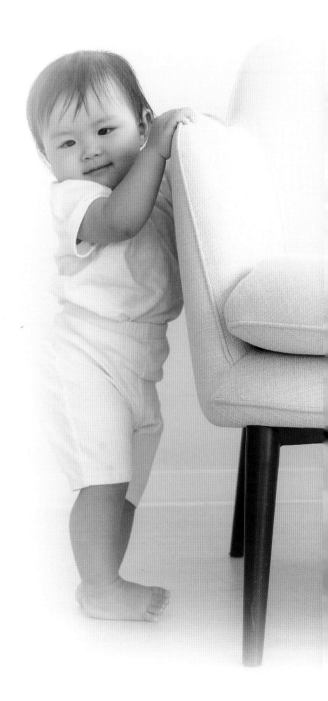

KEY BENEFITS OF SOFT GYMNASTICS

- Encourages your baby to develop and maintain suppleness, good muscle tone and joint flexibility.

- Encourages your baby to develop and maintain an open chest and shoulders, a strong back and good posture as they grow and strengthen.

- Builds up self-confidence and a good body image.

- Encourages structural symmetry and balance.

- Encourages your baby to maintain and develop abdominal breathing and muscular relaxation, both at rest and while in action.

- Encourages a more confident physical and emotional relationship with parents.

ENCOURAGING MOBILITY

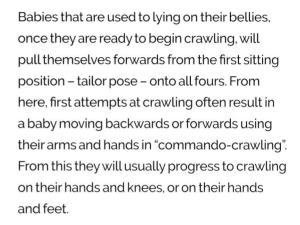

Although most babies will crawl for some time before they stand and walk properly, some stand and walk without crawling. Usually, if a baby misses the crawling phase it is because they have not spent enough waking time lying on their tummy and are more reticent about moving onto all fours. Such babies are often "bottom shufflers", and will move themselves around in a sitting position.

Babies that are used to lying on their bellies, once they are ready to begin crawling, will pull themselves forwards from the first sitting position – tailor pose – onto all fours. From here, first attempts at crawling often result in a baby moving backwards or forwards using their arms and hands in "commando-crawling". From this they will usually progress to crawling on their hands and knees, or on their hands and feet.

At the same time as your baby makes their early attempts at crawling, they will develop their second sitting position and may begin to stand with support. As they develop strength and confidence, they will start to pull themselves up from squatting to standing, with support, and practise lifting their legs. Once they are able to lift and lower one leg at a time, they will begin to enjoy walking sideways around furniture, and walking forwards holding your hands.

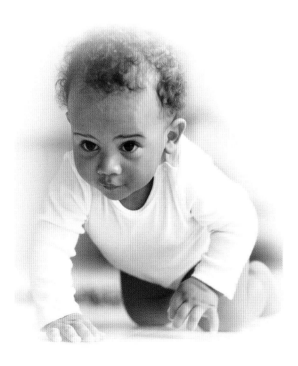

ENCOURAGING MOBILITY

PREPARING

Once your baby is sitting independently, kneel on the floor and sit them over your thigh. Let them squat and stand with their feet either side of your leg. This will help their feet to spread and their legs to strengthen. Let them bounce. Support them but don't lift them up.

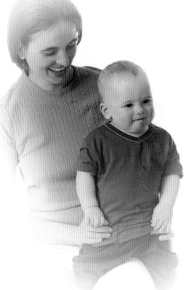

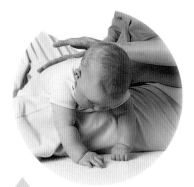

CRAWLING

To encourage your baby to crawl, rock them to and fro over your thigh, while they are in an all-fours position.

· Keep it fun!

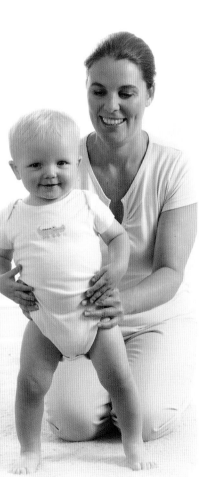

STANDING

Stand them on their feet and hold them by the waist. Bear down gently, giving them the weight of your hands for stronger roots and better balance. You can develop this by taking your hands to their hips and bearing down.

· Continue for as long as it's fun and your baby is comfortable.

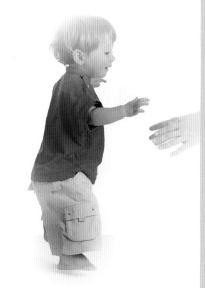

WALKING

Once your baby is standing, you can encourage them to walk. Sit on the floor, opposite your partner, friend or family member – you should be close enough to touch each other's outstretched hands. With your baby standing in between you, call their name to encourage them to walk between you.

· Continue for as long as you and your baby are having fun.

Tailor-pose swing

When most adults sit on the floor, they tend to curve their spines and their weight is supported by their lower backs. This sitting position is not only uncomfortable to maintain for any length of time, but it is also damaging to the back and the spine and can inhibit the functions of breathing and digestion.

By practising this swing, your baby will achieve the strength and flexibility necessary to enable them to continue to sit with their weight on the back of their thighs. This takes the strain off their lower back and maintains good sitting posture. Your baby's internal organs benefit because in this position their chest is open and their tummy is relaxed, allowing them to breathe more deeply and encouraging a more healthy digestive rhythm.

This position is also practical for your developing baby – by maintaining flexibility, their spine is free to bend from their hip joints, allowing them to reach forwards freely in all directions.

As your baby progresses from sitting to standing, they may lose some of their flexibility and with it, their perfect sitting posture. It is important, therefore, to keep using the tailor-pose swing to ensure that your child's hips remain flexible and that they retain a strong, straight back and good posture as they grow and develop.

The swing will soon become a game that your child will actively enjoy and look forward to – you may find that if you forget to do it, they will be quick to remind you.

*

If your baby is too heavy for you to lift, bounce them gently in this position on the top of a child's fitness (Gymnic) ball. Hold onto them securely at all times.

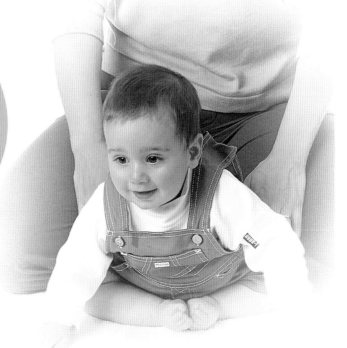

TAILOR-POSE SWING

1 Sit your baby on your lap in tailor pose with your arms under their arms and over their legs. Bring the soles of their feet together and gently pull them into the trunk of their body. Clap their feet together and slowly rock your baby from side to side.

• Continue for about 20 seconds.

2 Now raise yourself off your heels and support your baby by holding their ankles. Your baby will be held securely between your forearms.

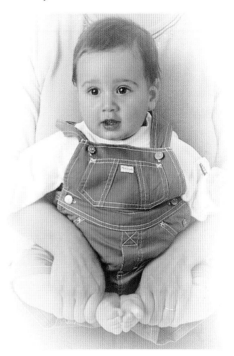

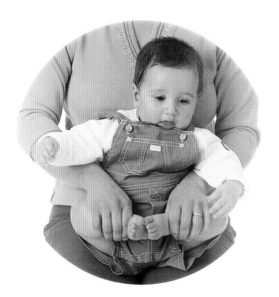

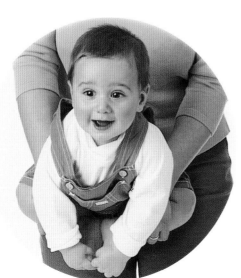

3 Now start to swing your baby gently from side to side. Do this five or six times – as your baby finds their rhythm they will relax and begin to enjoy it. Continue to swing and now let your baby lean forwards, taking their chest towards their feet. Make sure that your arms remain under your baby's arms throughout the exercise.

• Continue for 4–5 swings.

 Throughout this soft gymnastic game, make sure that your arms remain under your baby's arms and over their legs.

Strong, flexible legs

As the "roots" of the body, the legs must be strong enough to support and carry it yet supple enough to allow a wide range of movement when both sitting and standing, and jumping and running. When your baby begins to explore their range of movement and "finds their feet", they will become more confident and a little more independent.

As your baby's legs strengthen, they will no longer stand and walk with their legs and feet open "cowboy style" because their inside thigh muscles will contract and draw them in line with their hips. At the same time, other postural muscles – such as in the calves, front thighs and buttocks – will strengthen to make their legs more stable. If these muscles strengthen without being stretched, your baby can lose a degree of their body's range of movement. For example, they will no longer be able to take their foot to their face or enjoy the full freedom of movement in tailor pose.

Your baby has spent a great deal of time and effort establishing a wide range of movement and it makes good sense to help them to retain this as they gain strength. Playing these soft gymnastic games once or twice a week will ensure that your baby maintains flexible joints and continues to enjoy a wide variety of movement and good posture.

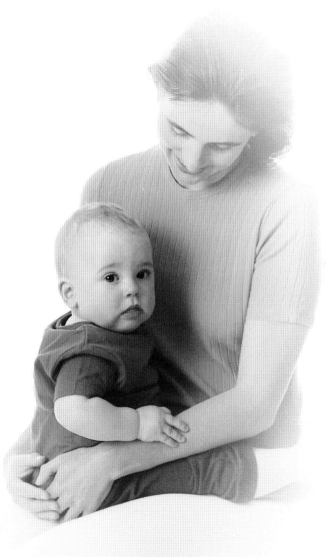

*

KEEPING HIPS FLEXIBLE
You can help to maintain your baby's hip flexibility by sitting with them so that their legs are outstretched around your waist.

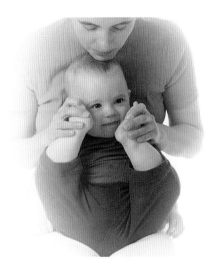

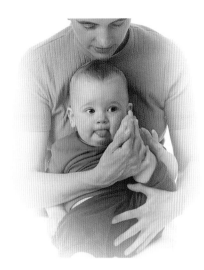

1 Sit your baby on your thighs and lean back slightly as you take your baby's feet to their face. Rock them from side to side and sing to them.

· Continue for about 30 seconds.

2 Hold one of your baby's legs from the back of the thigh and knee, and let the other leg straighten. Rub and massage the back of the thigh as you continue to rock and sing.

· Continue for 30 seconds. Repeat with his other leg.

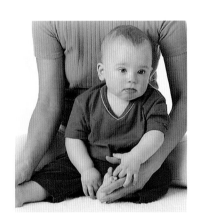

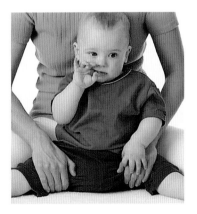

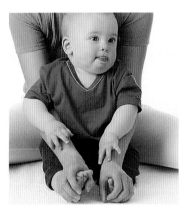

3 Let your baby sit between your knees in "side splits" – with their legs and feet open. Close one leg in a half tailor pose, then straighten it and close the other.

· Repeat this movement from leg to leg rhythmically for about 30 seconds.

4 As your baby sits upright, open both of their legs. Rock them while you gently massage their inner thighs.

· Continue for 20–30 seconds.

5 Gently bring your baby's legs together and, keeping their legs straight, extend their heels by taking their feet in your hands then turning them out.

· Hold for a few seconds.

An open chest and shoulders

Unlike adults, who usually restrict their breathing to their chests and inhibit their emotional expressions to facial and hand movements, a child expresses themselves with their whole body – jumping up and down and throwing open their arms with delight or shaking their fists and stamping their feet with rage. Babies are active; their responses are spontaneous and their breathing rhythm is full and easy.

Young children have an intuitive understanding of the intimate relationship between feeling, breathing and movement.

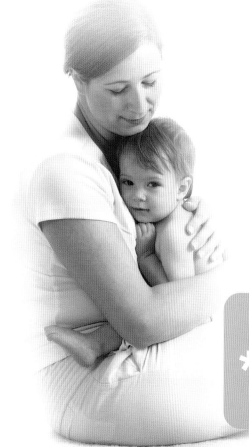

As well as expressing their emotions with uninhibited movement, to suppress feeling – to subdue fear or acute anxiety – they will make themselves motionless, become very still and hold their breath.

Observe how your baby sits and stands; their straight back, free chest and relaxed shoulders reveal a positive attitude to life and a state of mind untainted by negativity. Watch how your baby breathes; every breath descends deep into their belly and their chest and abdomen work in harmony – expanding and contracting together.

Your baby's straight back and their open chest and shoulders illustrate the structural balance of their posture, where weight is easily carried and transferred bone upon bone without undue stress being placed upon the muscles. This allows the muscles to function healthily and to retain a high degree of relaxation, even when the body is mobile.

Even from an early age, babies enjoy arching their backs and it is this intuitive movement that contributes greatly to the healthy nature of their posture and breathing rhythms.

> ### EXTENDING THE SPINE
> Try this with your child lying back over a children's fitness ball. Start from a standing position and, once you and your child are both confident, bounce them very gently – and keep it fun!

*

AN OPEN CHEST AND SHOULDERS

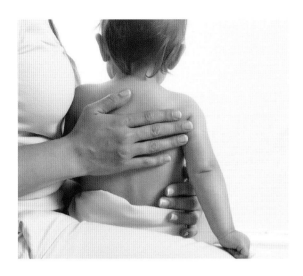

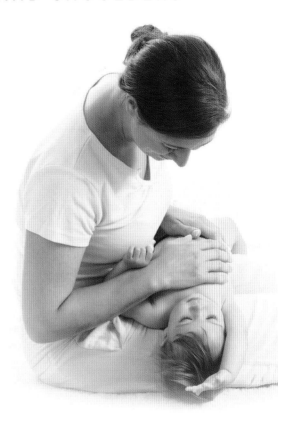

1 Sit on the floor against a wall or on the edge of a cushion with your legs straight. When you are comfortable, sit your baby across your lap, so that they are facing to one side.

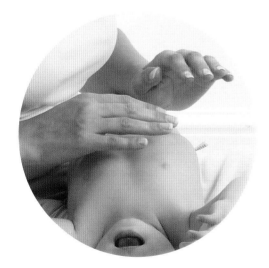

2 Now lay your baby back over your thighs, so that their feet remain on the floor and their head and back are arched. To encourage this movement, rock your baby gently and slowly roll your legs from side to side while you sing to them.

3 Once your baby is relaxed in this position, pat their chest with cupped hands, rub their belly clockwise and stroke down the front of their thighs. Keep rolling your legs gently as you continue this light massage.

• Continue for about 30 seconds.

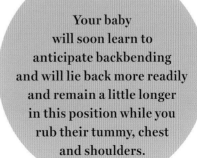

*
Your baby
will soon learn to
anticipate backbending
and will lie back more readily
and remain a little longer
in this position while you
rub their tummy, chest
and shoulders.

Body confidence and agility

Children engage in vigorous physical games and activities that often demand a wide range of physical movement. The flexibility of the spine and the strength of the muscles that support it are therefore of great importance.

Once they can stand, your child must secure their balance and will continually test the boundaries of their movements and the potential abilities of their body. This will undoubtedly involve the odd tumble or two, but because children are more relaxed than adults – both in action and at rest – the shock of impact when they fall generally passes right through their bodies.

You can engage your baby in the following soft gymnastic game once they are on their feet and continue for as long as you can lift them and you both enjoy it. Practised once or twice a week, it will encourage agility and self confidence. Once your child "gets

the feel" of this exercise they will demand endless repetition. This can be a lot of fun for you both and encourage more trust in your relationship. The confidence that we feel in being supported or grounded from the hips downwards we mostly take for granted. This "tumbling" exercise reinforces that feeling every time your child turns and lands on their feet. Ensure that your hands are over their shoulders and on the inner side of their arms as you stand up on your knees to roll them backwards.

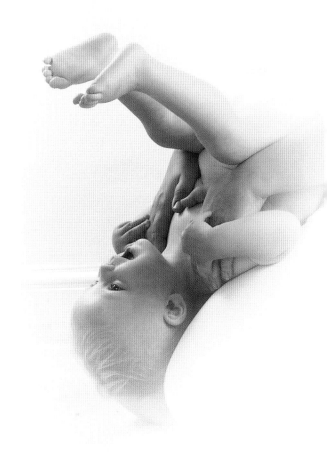

*

DUAL-PURPOSE ACTIVITY

This is also a trust game and one in which your baby's world first turns upside-down before they centres themselves.

BODY CONFIDENCE AND AGILITY

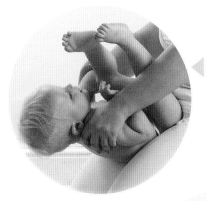

1 Kneeling comfortably on your feet on a cushion, sit your baby on your lap, facing you, belly-to-belly.

2 Now, holding their legs securely around the sides of your body under your arms, place both of your hands on their back – one at the base of their neck, the other around their lower back, across their hips. Let your baby lean backwards and gently open their chest and shoulders by pushing their upper back. Talk, sing and rock them gently, keeping them fully engaged.

• Continue for about 20 seconds.

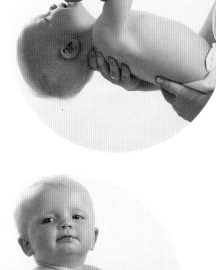

3 Now, lower your baby and let them lean back over your knees, and place your hands over their shoulders. Rock your thighs gently from side to side to relax your baby.

• Continue for about 20 seconds.

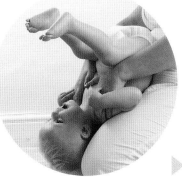
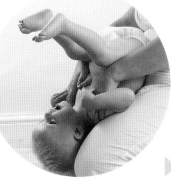

4 Your hands must be on the insides of your baby's arms. Making sure that your baby's legs can roll unimpeded, stand up on your knees, supporting them from over their shoulders, and let them roll backwards through your arms.

5 When they have landed in a standing position, drop your hands down, hold them from around the hips and bear down gently using just the weight of your hands to "ground" them.

REINTRODUCING MASSAGE

Increasing mobility and the urge to explore generally mean that most babies go through a period during which they resist lying still long enough for an "all-over" massage. When this happens, don't undress your baby for massage, but whenever you are sitting together, continue to rub their back and their head and feet. Try to maintain this kind of affectionate touch whenever it is mutually enjoyable. Although your baby may not want to be undressed and massaged, the need to be held and touched is still tremendously important; your sustained physical reassurances will continue to add to your child's sense of self-worth and healthy body image. Lots of spontaneous hugs, kisses and strokes will add to your baby's self-esteem and make it easier for you to reintroduce massage into your relationship. When you feel the time is right, usually around 18 months, try to introduce the following routine in your child's time rather than yours. This is usually when they are at their most relaxed – for example, before their afternoon nap or bedtime – but not on an empty or full tummy.

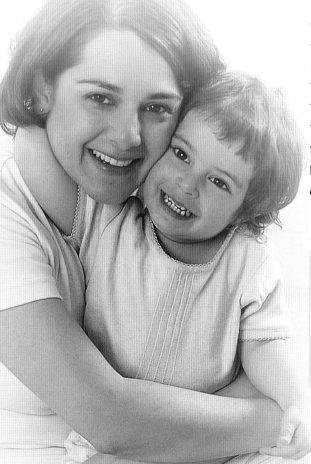

CONTINUED CLOSENESS
The need to be held and to be touched continues throughout life. Maintain enjoyable physical contact with your child as they grow and develop.

REINTRODUCING MASSAGE

A stronger touch

The onset of the "terrible twos", from about 18 months, is the time your baby begins to assert themselves and their quest for independence, and requires even more patience and understanding on your part. Appropriately, it seems that around this age there are periods when babies once again enjoy being massaged and these interludes can often provide a welcome break in the emotional extremes that may prevail at this time.

Now that your baby is stronger and more resilient, you may need to add more depth to your touch and give a slightly stronger and faster massage. To keep your baby's attention, you must continue to talk, sing and maintain eye contact with your child as much as you can, for as long as you massage. This is the time to teach your child the vital skill of breathing out whenever you ask them to calm down. A deep exhalation can relax the body and quieten the mind. It's a wonderful skill that will serve them well in years to come.

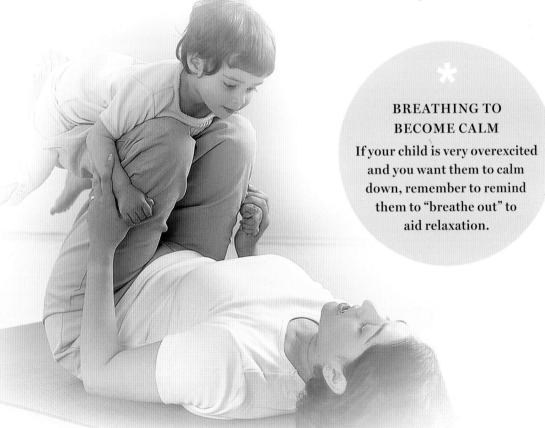

*

BREATHING TO BECOME CALM

If your child is very overexcited and you want them to calm down, remember to remind them to "breathe out" to aid relaxation.

REINTRODUCING MASSAGE

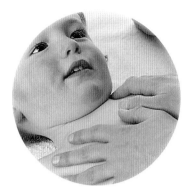

1 Place both hands on the centre of your child's chest and massage upwards, outwards and back to the centre with your relaxed hands.

• Repeat 4–5 times.

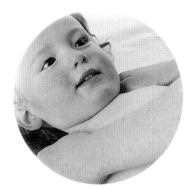

2 Rub your child's shoulders gently but firmly backwards and forwards from the sides of their neck outwards.

• Continue for about 20 seconds.

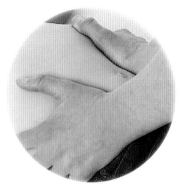

3 Keeping your hands on your child's skin, stroke downwards from the shoulders to the hips and back again.

• Repeat 4–5 times.

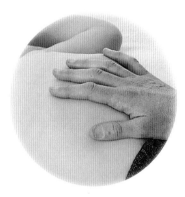

4 Using the relaxed weight of one hand, massage your child's belly clockwise in a circular motion.

• Repeat 5–6 times.

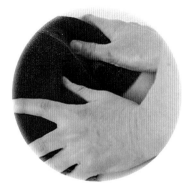

5 Massage the front of your child's thighs by squeezing and releasing and rubbing gently five or six times then slide your hands to their calves and repeat the movements.

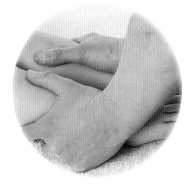

6 Keep your hands on your child's skin and stroke back up to their shoulders and right down to their feet.

• Repeat 3–4 times, ending with the feet.

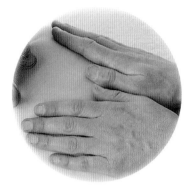

7 With your child lying on their belly, rub their shoulders with your palms and massage the sides of their upper spine, pressing in gently with your thumbs.

· Continue for about 20 seconds.

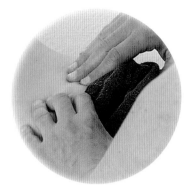

8 Stroke down your baby's back from their shoulders to their feet, using the relaxed weight of both hands. Using your fingertips, massage the base of their spine and rub gently.

· Repeat 3–4 times.

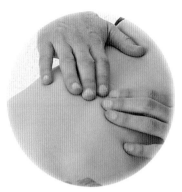

9 With the middle fingers and index fingers of both hands, glide up both sides of your baby's back from the base of the spine to the back of the neck and back down again.

· Continue for about 20 seconds.

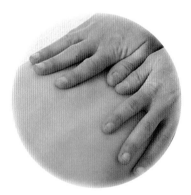

10 Now spread your fingers and draw the relaxed weight of your hands all the way down to the feet. Glide your hands back up to the base of your baby's spine.

· Repeat 3–4 times.

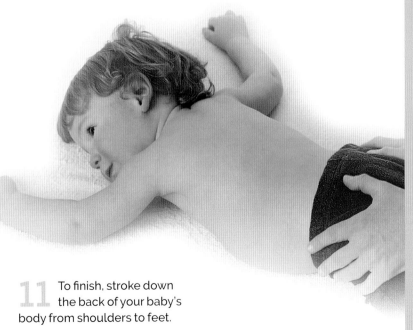

11 To finish, stroke down the back of your baby's body from shoulders to feet.

· Repeat 3–4 times.

THERAPEUTIC TOUCH FOR SICKNESS AND ADDITIONAL NEEDS

Many childhood ailments and illnesses render the skin hypersensitive and "prickly" and when your baby is distinctly unwell, they will not want to be massaged in the normal way. Quite often what a baby most wants and needs is to sleep and be held until the prescribed remedy becomes effective. In instances like this, when you find yourself lying or sitting comfortably with your baby, try gently squeezing and kneading their hands and feet and stroking their head lightly with your fingertips – these techniques are non-invasive and can be relaxing and comforting.

The same approach can be used if your baby is emotionally upset, if they do not respond well to touch, find it difficult to relax and let go when being held, and cry easily.

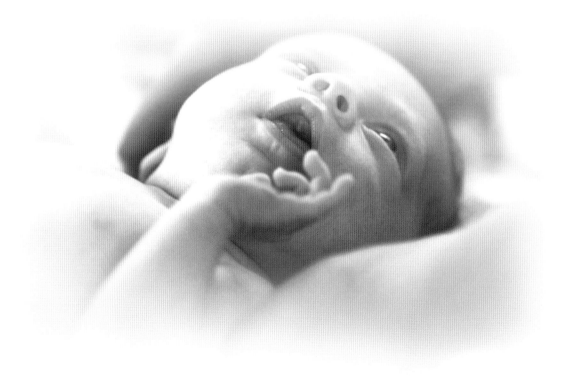

THERAPEUTIC TOUCH FOR SICKNESS AND ADDITIONAL NEEDS

In the following chapter are some techniques for more specific conditions, but none of these are meant to be used as a substitute for professional diagnosis and recommendations.

Babies with additional needs can also benefit from massage and you can modify techniques or bring out certain elements of massage to suit particular needs.

KEY BENEFITS OF THERAPEUTIC TOUCH TECHNIQUES

- Soothe common childhood complaints.

- Can comfort a generally fractious child.

- Help you to combat various types of congestion.

- Enable parents to ease physical and emotional problems.

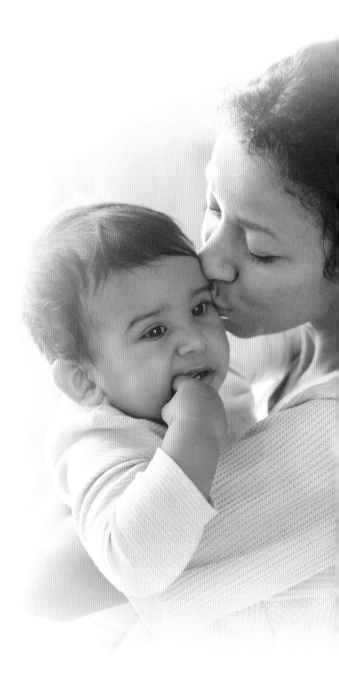

Coughs, colds and congestion

A young baby will only breathe through their mouth when their nostrils are completely blocked with mucus. In the daytime, this may not cause too much of a problem, but at night it can prove to be a major source of discomfort. When your baby sleeps, their breathing rhythm becomes slower and deeper and if their nostrils are congested, they will gasp for air and awake with a start. This can be quite disruptive, particularly if your baby has already established a sleeping routine.

If your baby is congested, place them in a more upright position when they are sleeping. You can do this by raising one end of their cot by securely placing a book or telephone directory underneath – don't let your baby sleep on a pillow. And avoid giving them mucus-making foods, such as dairy products.

These techniques will show you how to relieve nostril and chest congestion, but they are not meant as a substitute for a professional diagnosis and treatment, rather as an aid to your baby's recovery. You may want to try the technique for freeing blocked nostrils on yourself first, before using it on your baby.

FREEING BLOCKED NOSTRILS

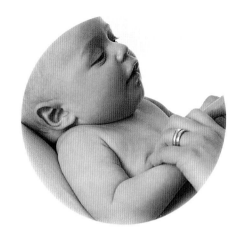

1 Sit on the floor with your back resting against a wall and your knees raised. Put your baby on your lap so that they are facing you.

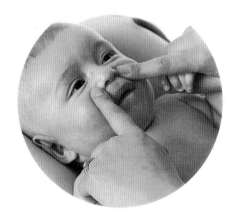

2 Gently press your index fingertips into each side of your baby's nostrils and draw the nostrils open by pressing gently downwards and outwards under the cheekbones.

· Repeat 4–5 times.

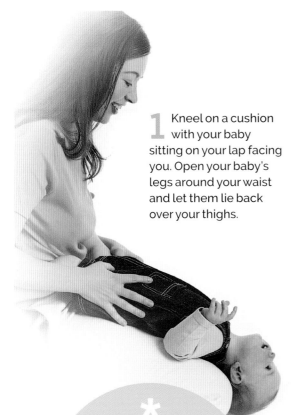

1 Kneel on a cushion with your baby sitting on your lap facing you. Open your baby's legs around your waist and let them lie back over your thighs.

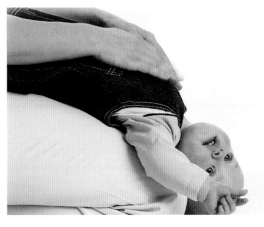

2 Using the relaxed weight of your cupped hands, pat all around the centre, and then the sides, of your baby's chest.

· Continue for about 30 seconds.

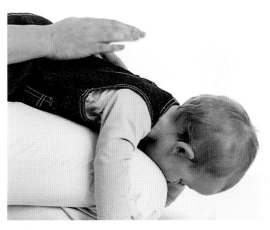

3 Now, place your baby on your thighs so they lie forwards on their belly and, using the relaxed weight of your cupped hands, pat all around their back and sides. If your baby is heavily congested, they may vomit slightly following this percussion movement, as the bronchial tubes compress and expel the mucus.

· Continue for about 30 seconds.

*
Some essential oils, such as eucalyptus and lavender, are recommended for clearing the sinuses. Mix 2 drops of the essential oil into 3 tablespoons of your base oil.

! Do not use essential oils for babies under 12 weeks. Eucalyptus will cancel any benefits of homeopathic treatment.

Relieving sticky eye

It is not uncommon for babies to have sticky eyes in the first day or two of life – usually as a result of amniotic fluid and other secretions entering the eyes at birth – and this stickiness usually disappears spontaneously. Beyond the first 48 hours, however, a sticky eye is due to infection. Otherwise known as conjunctivitis, a red and sticky eye often clears if you cleanse the eye with a cotton wool swab and some tepid boiled water – gently wiping outwards from the inside corners. If redness and stickiness persist, medical advice should be sought.

An eye that is continuously sticky and watery can be due to a blocked tear duct. The tear ducts are lined with mucous membrane, an extension of that which lines the nostrils. When this membrane becomes inflamed and swollen, the tear ducts become blocked, causing tears to flow from the eyes rather than drain into the nose as they usually do. Try this simple technique to clear the blockage.

Do not use oil for this technique as it can enter your baby's eye. Make sure that your hands are clean and that your fingernails cannot scratch your baby.

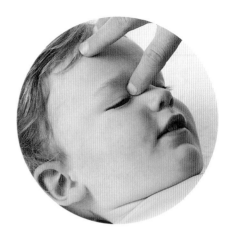

1 The tear glands and ducts are located in the depression in the nasal bone in the corner of the eye and run down the side of the bridge of the nose. Place your index finger outside the corner of your baby's eye and press gently into the side of the nose. You may need to steady your baby's head with your free hand while you do this.

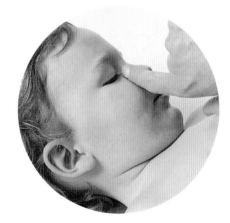

2 Draw your finger downwards, along the side of your baby's nostril and under the cheekbone.

· Repeat 3–4 times.

Treating glue ear

If your baby has any ear discharge, other than wax, or appears to be in pain, consult your doctor immediately. This could be a middle ear infection that needs immediate medical attention.

Glue ear refers to the discharge of a thick, sticky substance in the middle ear, which prevents the eardrum from moving normally and can cause partial deafness. This chronic condition is often the result of recurrent episodes of acute otitis media (middle ear infection).

Glue ear can sometimes be treated by a competent cranial osteopath but, as a preventive measure, try the following sequence when you massage your baby's head and neck. You may wish to use some oil to make the movement smoother.

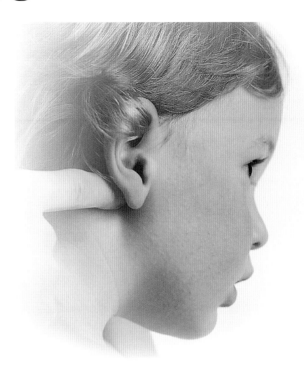

1 With your baby facing away from you, place your index fingers on the side of their head, behind the lobes of their ears.

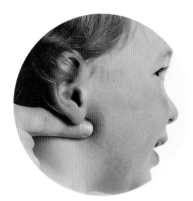

2 Press your fingers gently into the sides of your baby's upper jawbone, behind their ears, and draw them downwards around the edge of the jawbone towards their throat.

• Repeat 3–4 times.

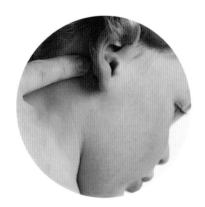

3 Now, press your index fingers again behind the lobes of both of your baby's ears and gently draw them downwards and towards you, around the sides and base of the skull.

• Repeat 3–4 times.

Wind, colic and constipation

We all take in air while we are eating and drinking, but because of the immaturity of your young baby's digestive system, air in the stomach or intestines can result in an uncomfortable pocket of gas. Wind is more common in bottle-fed babies so the first thing to check is that the hole in the teat is neither too small nor too large – the formula should drip out at a steady flow of one drop per second. Also ensure that the bottle is tilted and that the milk completely fills the teat. If not, this will result in your baby taking in too much air with their milk. Try to keep your baby's back straight while feeding and when they have finished, pat them between the shoulder blades and stroke their back from the bottom to the top, while tilting them forwards slightly.

No one really knows what causes colic – long spells of crying that usually occur at night – and there are no certain cures, but if you are breastfeeding, eating wholesome, nourishing foods regularly and giving yourself time to eat properly, these may help. It is also not uncommon for breastfed babies to go for a few days occasionally without emptying their bowels. Giving your baby plenty of waking time on their belly (see page 18) can prevent and relieve reflux, colic and constipation as this position stretches and relaxes the abdomen, but do not do this immediately after a feed – let them digest their food first.

You also can use tummy massage but not when your baby is distressed – try the Tiger in the Tree (see pages 88–89) instead. The techniques here can be used between bouts of discomfort, when your baby is neither too hungry nor too full. A good opportunity for this massage is during a nappy change.

*

SOFTEN THE BELLY

If your baby's belly is hard and unyielding, gently move their hands out of the way then gently lay your relaxed hand across the belly before you begin to massage.

WIND, COLIC AND CONSTIPATION

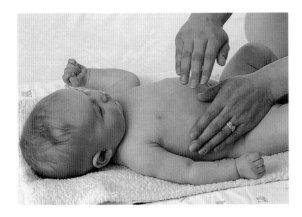 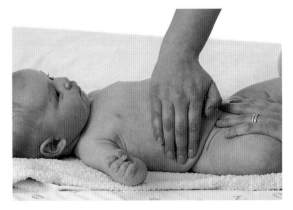

1 Lay your baby on the floor and, using the relaxed weight of your whole hand, massage hand-over-hand down the right side of their abdomen, from between the hip and the lower rib across to below the navel.

· Continue for 2–3 minutes and then repeat on the left side of your baby's abdomen.

2 Cup your hand and place it horizontally across your baby's belly. Squeeze gently and knead the belly from side to side. Don't push downwards or your baby will resist and tense up. Keep it gentle and playful, so that their belly softens.

· Continue for about 20 seconds.

3 Now, using the relaxed weight of your cupped hand, massage your baby's belly with your hand and the tummy moving in a circular motion clockwise from your left to your right.

· Repeat 4–5 times.

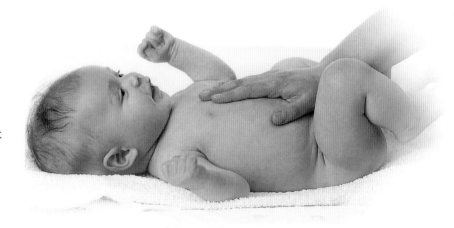

! If your baby is suffering from wind, colic or constipation, consult your doctor and, if necessary, a nutritionist to rule out the possibility that your baby is allergic to something in their diet or, if you are breastfeeding, to something in yours. When all else fails use Tiger in the Tree (see pages 88–89) and try more tummy time (see pages 18–19).

Teething and irritability

Teething starts some weeks before your baby's teeth make an appearance, which can be any time between three and twelve months. The first tooth is usually the lower central incisor and, following this, seven other incisors appear – four upper and four lower incisors altogether – enabling your baby to bite. In all, your child will cut 20 milk, or baby, teeth – as opposed to 32 permanent teeth, which will start to appear when they are about six years of age.

There are many symptoms incorrectly attributed to teething such as fever, diarrhoea, poor appetite, vomiting, coughing and a runny nose. As any of these could be the result of a serious illness, if your baby appears to be unwell, seek professional advice.

Most teeth erupt without any detectable pain or discomfort but in the day or two before or after eruption, your baby may exhibit some fussiness, drooling and a desire to chomp on a hard object. If your baby suffers discomfort, a hard, cold object – such as a gel-filled teething ring – may provide relief. If your baby is experiencing particular distress, massaging their hands, feet and back is non-intrusive and can comfort them when they are restless and upset.

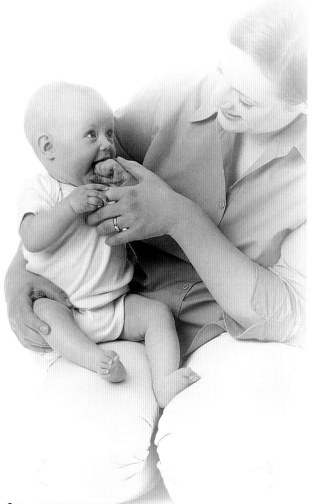

SIGNS OF TEETHING

Some babies salivate and press their hands into their mouths when they are teething.

TEETHING AND IRRITABILITY

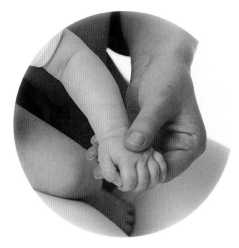

1 Sitting with your baby on your lap, squeeze and stroke their hands gently between your thumb and fingers.

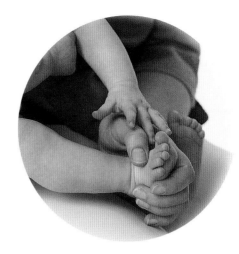

2 Take the massage down to your baby's feet, squeezing gently and stroking both the tops and the soles of their feet.

3 Now, hold your baby close and stroke them gently all over their back and up and down the length of their spine. Talk to them softly as you massage them.

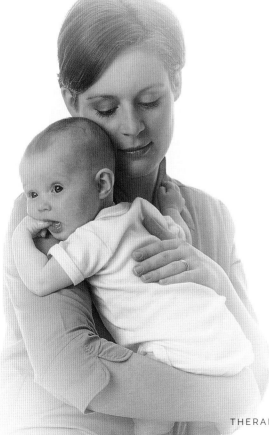

*

A natural remedy such as chamomile roman can be effective for soothing your baby during teething. Dilute a few drops in full-fat milk and pour this into your baby's bath.

Sleeplessness

Most young babies do not sleep through the night. Your baby has been close to you for nine months so to expect them to conform to a routine in a new and unfamiliar environment is unrealistic. A young baby needs feeding fairly often so your baby cannot help but interrupt your sleep to be fed. Once fed and changed, your baby should return to sleep after a cuddle. Remember that physical contact is vital for babies, and a little time spent in your arms is often all that is needed for your baby to settle. (Tiger in the Tree is deeply relaxing, see pages 88–89.)

After your baby has settled into a longer sleep routine they may still resist going to bed and, when awakened, returning back to sleep. If your baby is not hungry or uncomfortable and stops crying while they are in your arms but cries when you try to lay them down, the following technique could be extremely useful. It will allow you to withdraw gradually, to offer your baby a loving touch that will reassure them of your presence and induce tranquillity and sleep.

Much of the success of this technique will depend on you positioning yourself comfortably, persevering and being consistent. Once your baby has accepted it, you will find that the technique will induce sleep, and that your baby will begin to anticipate it.

The same technique can be used when you feel that the time is right to introduce a routine and put your baby to bed at a regular hour. You can begin to withdraw further by shortening the time spent stroking but leaving your hands on your baby until they are asleep. When you have established this, you can reduce the time still further and remove your hands when your baby is almost asleep – but remain within sight of them and quietly reassure them. If your baby is able to sit and sits up crying, gently lie them down and continue. The final step is to lie your baby down, stroke them, tell them it's time to sleep and slowly withdraw.

*

NIGHT-TIME ROUTINE

Using this simple technique and a little patience, you will help your baby to drift off to sleep.

SLEEPLESSNESS

1 Start by laying your baby on their side; you can always turn them onto their back once they are asleep. Stroke around the top of their back or head using the relaxed weight of your whole hand.

2 Then stroke down the length of their back in the same way as you would a puppy or a kitten.

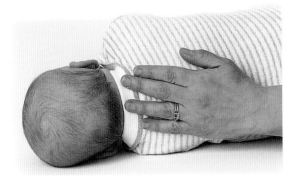

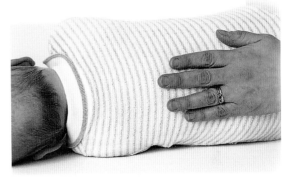

3 Place a relaxed hand across your baby's head, which fits perfectly into the palm of your hand and your fingers.

4 Keeping one hand on you baby's head, place a relaxed hand across your baby's tummy and knead the tummy very gently from side to side. As your baby relaxes, this will induce feelings of tranquillity. Withdraw very slowly once your baby is sleeping.

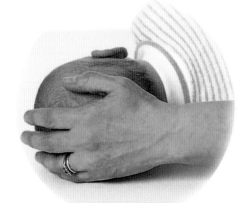

! Do not leave your baby to "cry it out". Persevere with this technique as a crying baby separated from their parent has high levels of stress hormones and this is not good for babies (or for parents).

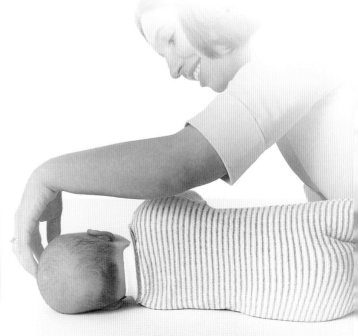

TIGER IN THE TREE

Tiger in the Tree is a wonderful position in which you can hold and massage your baby from birth to relax their tummy and relieve birth trauma, colic, wind, constipation, fractiousness, anxiety and other ailments associated with acute abdominal tension.

The technique is both curative and preventative – it can be used on the spot to bring instant relief to your baby when they need it most, as well as on a daily basis to help them develop a cumulative sense of ease that can dramatically improve their whole disposition. It won't work, however, if your baby is hungry.

The tummy is an emotional centre and a great source of tranquillity. Keep your baby's tummy relaxed and you will keep your baby relaxed. Having them lie forwards in your arms, combined with gentle side-to-side abdominal massage, initiates a deep sense of relief and relaxation that pervades their entire body. Supporting your baby on both of your arms allows you to sustain the position for a longer period of time, so that your baby enjoys the maximum effect of the massage.

Fathers, especially, will find this is a useful technique because the baby is facing away from the breast and will not add to their tummy discomfort by trying to feed. It also gives fathers a successful position in which to soothe a distressed baby.

The way in which you hold and massage your baby is essential to the success of this technique. Maintain your own sense of relaxation by keeping your shoulders and hands relaxed and your exhalation deep and breathing rhythmic. Take your time and rock, talk or sing softly and your baby will sense your calmness and adapt to you, rather than you becoming upset and adapting to them.

This technique can be practised with your baby naked or clothed. Its effects are immediate and it can be performed anywhere and at any time. Your baby does not need to be upset to practise this technique. Get them used to this position. The more you practise, the easier it gets and the greater the benefits.

TIGER IN THE TREE

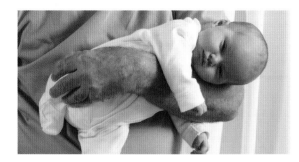

1 Hold your baby with their back to you and bring your left arm across your baby's chest, taking care to drop their left arm under yours so that you can comfortably cradle their head and neck in the crook of your elbow.

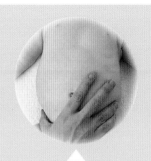

INTERNAL ORGANS

With your hand spread, your thumb is on the ascending colon and your fingers are on the descending colon (both between the lower ribs and hips).

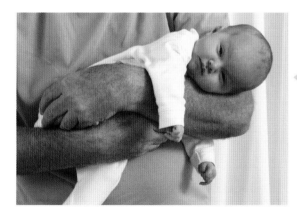

2 Bring your right hand between your baby's knees and place your palm across your baby's tummy, supporting them equally in both of your arms. Tuck your baby's foot into the crook of your arm, turn them over onto your hand and rock them gently from the hip.

3 As they lie belly forwards over your hand, very gently knead their tummy from side to side with your relaxed hand. The weight of their body as it lies on your working hand adds to the efficiency of the massage as you are able to attain deeper contact without pressing in. If, after a few minutes, your baby continues to experience discomfort, walk them around in this position and gently pat their lower chest.

• Repeat this technique frequently and try to establish the position as a regular holding position.

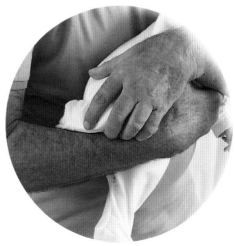

Caesarean babies

Babies delivered by elective Caesarean section with a total absence of labour miss the protracted contractions that accompany a normal delivery, and which stimulate the baby's peripheral nervous system and principal organs of survival. Consequently, these babies will benefit even more from a regular massage. As well as all the conventional benefits, a regular period of time spent massaging your baby also will give you the opportunity to strengthen your emotional attachments. Attempts at bonding may have been difficult at your baby's birth because of the medical attention required immediately after surgery and because your body needs time to recover; physical closeness can be made more difficult by your inability to lift and carry your baby while your body is healing.

Following a Caesarean section, you can use some of your recovery period to lie with your baby and introduce the massage routine for the very young baby (see pages 10–15). By the time your baby is ready to move on to a more formal routine, you should be more able to lift and carry them. Until your scar has healed, it is best not to do anything that puts pressure on your lower abdomen. Once you feel able to lift and carry your baby, keep your arms as close to your body as you can. Never try to lift them at arm's length, as this will

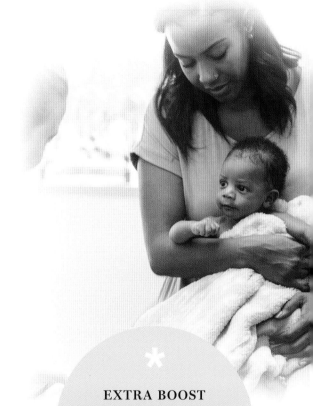

* EXTRA BOOST

Once your scar has healed, "tummy time" will provide the same benefits for you as it does for your baby.

place enormous strain on your lower back and belly. Caesarean babies can be more prone to lethargy, so massaging your baby will give them the stimulation that they need, as well as the opportunity for you to check and promote their structural health and engage with them emotionally.

Premature babies

Given the high quality and sophistication of current neonatal care, most premature babies – including some weighing as little as 900 grams – survive. Very premature babies can be hyper-sensitive to touch and have their heart rates, body temperatures and blood pressures constantly monitored within a sterile incubator. Because of these conditions, touching and stroking can be difficult, but you can still make contact with the most accessible parts of your baby's body, starting with hands and feet.

A baby who spends a long period of time in an incubator can associate touch with medical procedures and may cry when handled. But a parent's touch is super beneficial and skin-to-skin contact once you are able to hold your child is known to regulate a premature baby's heartbeat, breathing rhythm and body temperature. So touch your baby and – when and where possible – hold and handle them to engage in as much skin-to-skin contact as is possible, both in the hospital and at home. This includes nappy changing and bathing.

Premature babies miss valuable "womb time" so are given a corrected age, which is the chronological age minus the number of weeks or months they were early. In my experience, however, a baby born at 36 weeks on reaching 40 weeks is still not as developed as a baby born at 40 weeks, so it is useful to subtract half the missed "womb time" again from the corrected age to account for the additional loss of nourishment from the womb.

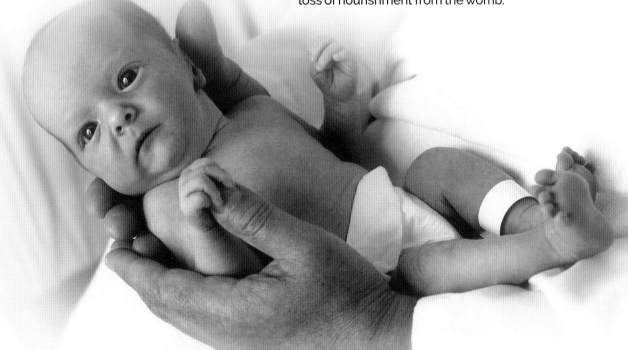

Visual impairments

Children with a visual impairment can benefit greatly from a regular massage. Perhaps even more than most babies, these children have a profound need for tactile stimulation. The sense of touch can provide a means of communication that allows the child to receive sensory information about their external world and a means to interact with it.

The impairment of one sense often leads to the greater development of another and this is especially true of touch. Children who are visually impaired depend upon their sense of touch to give form and recognition to the objects in their external world. Given regularly, massage can bring you more in touch with your child. This can make it easier for you to

Some babies with hearing or visual impairments may be slow to crawl and walk, possibly because they are more resistant to lying on their bellies as they feel cut off from what is around them. Introduce tummy time, slowly and early. When you massage your baby's back, try laying them supported on a cushion from the waist up.

guide them towards the objects they will use in their everyday life. It will also help them to overcome any resistance they may have to being touched and encourage them to be more socially interactive.

When you introduce massage, it is important to do it slowly. Begin by stroking your baby gently – talk to them and be attentive to their response. One mother I knew would close her eyes when she massaged her child. She would talk and sing and maintain a wealth of physical contact – stroking, kissing and keeping her face very close to her baby's.

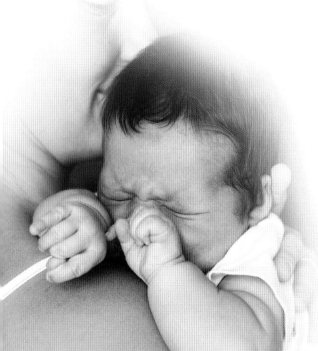

STIMULATING THE OTHER SENSES
To engage senses such as hearing and smell, talk softly and try to keep cheek-to-cheek with your baby as you introduce massage.

Hearing impairments

Babies with hearing impediments will benefit from massage. Given regularly, massage will encourage your baby's development and help you to appreciate the ways in which they communicate. This will strengthen your emotional relationship and add to your child's self-esteem. A baby who has a hearing impairment needs to be talked to and given lots of visual cues, as well as plenty of physical expressions of affection. Speak to your baby and mouth the words clearly as you say them, so that your baby can focus on you fully.

Introduce massage slowly and gently to overcome any initial tactile resistance. Stroke your baby and maintain eye contact as you explain what you are doing as you do it. Keep the massage enjoyable and pay close attention to your baby's response.

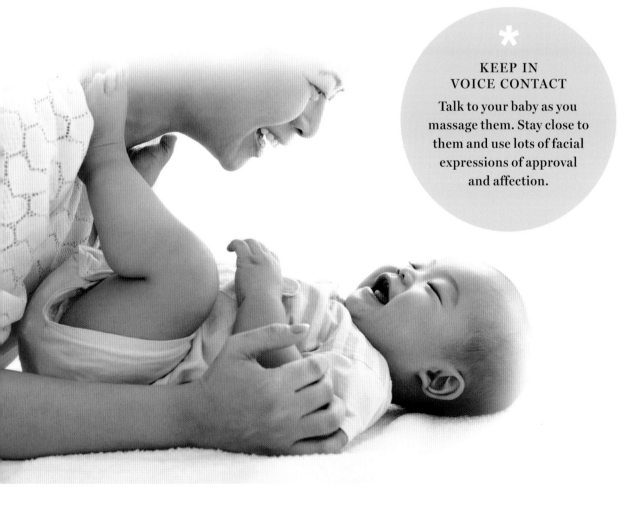

*
KEEP IN
VOICE CONTACT
Talk to your baby as you massage them. Stay close to them and use lots of facial expressions of approval and affection.

Talipes

This is a congenital deformity in a baby's foot or feet, which twists the foot out of shape or position. One of the most common forms of talipes is where the baby's foot turns inwards, often as a result of their position in the womb. This can be mild or severe and can sometimes be rectified by physiotherapy or if not, by a minor surgical procedure.

To straighten the baby's foot, the heel must extend. For the heel to do so, the calf muscle must relax and stretch to allow the movement. Here are some massage techniques that you can use, but check with your physiotherapist before you begin, and show them what you plan to do.

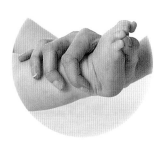

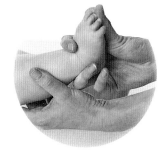

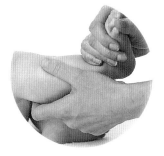

1 Kneeling comfortably on your feet on a cushion, pull your baby's lower leg and foot hand-over-hand through your palms. With your thumb turned downwards, draw your hand down your baby's calf. Follow through and turn the foot outwards to extend the heel as far as it will allow – without using any force.

2 Hold the foot in this position while you massage your baby's calf with your other hand.

• Continue for a few minutes or as long as your baby will allow. Repeat twice a day – morning and evening.

3 Now hold your baby's foot in the same position as you stroke and stimulate the muscle on the side of their shin with your fingertips.

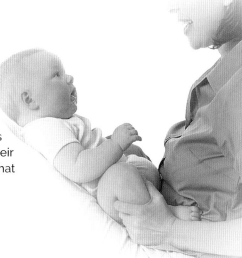

4 Sitting with your back supported, raise your knees and let your baby sit on your belly with their back resting against your knees. Their knees should be flexed and open with their feet resting against your chest or waist. Massage your baby's calf while simultaneously trying to extend the heel by pressing their foot against your chest or waist. Make sure you support them so that they cannot propel themselves over your knees.

• Continue for a few minutes or as long as your baby will allow. Repeat morning and night.

Cerebral palsy

This condition is attributed to a lack of development of the part of the brain concerned with movement and posture. Learning and visual difficulties including poor speech, hearing and vision may also be present if adjoining parts of the brain are also affected. The effects vary from child to child and range from slight to severe.

There are three recognized forms of cerebral palsy: ataxia – an unsteady walk with balancing difficulties; spasticity – disordered control of movement mostly associated with stiff muscles; and athetosis – uncontrollable or involuntary movements of different parts of the body.

The brain is "neuro plastic" and this brings with it the ability for change. And on a day-to-day basis, massage can bring a moderate-to-high degree of relief and an improvement in the quality of the child's daily life. Any improvement in muscle tone brings with it more potential for movement and can influence posture. Massage can help mobility. It can relieve the cramps that result from stiff muscles and can ease the chronic wind and constipation often associated with poor posture and the lack of movement. Circulation can be enhanced and a regular period of one-to-one physical contact through the medium of massage can be mutually enjoyable and improve communication between you.

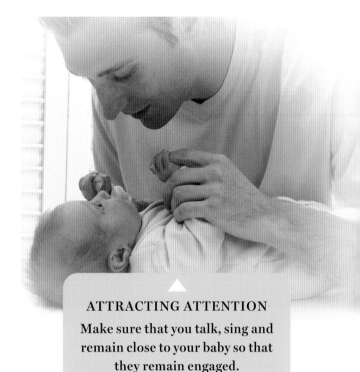

ATTRACTING ATTENTION
Make sure that you talk, sing and remain close to your baby so that they remain engaged.

Cerebral palsy can go unrecognized for the first year or more, so if you have reason to believe that your child may be affected, seek early intervention. If your baby has been diagnosed as suffering from this condition, the sooner you begin to massage them, the better. Obviously, never try to force open or closed any of your baby's joints – modify the techniques to suit your baby. If your baby resists being naked, massage them clothed. Introduce the massage slowly – maybe one part of your baby's body at a time, starting with their legs and feet and working up towards the head. Try to massage your baby daily and if you encounter any difficulties, consult your physiotherapist.

Index and acknowledgments

Acknowledgments

Thank you to all the mums, dads and babies who helped with the photography for this project.